OUR HORMONES,
OUR HEALTH

Dr Susanne Esche-Belke is a specialist in general medicine, and has been combining conventional medical knowledge with the latest findings in stress and integrative medicine in clinics and in her own practice for 20 years. Her focus is on the holistic therapy of female hormone and immune disorders. She is the co-founder of the women's health platform *Less — Doctors for Balance*.

Dr Suzann Kirschner-Brouns is a doctor and mediator. As a medical journalist and author, she writes on health issues for well-known publishers and magazines. Formerly editor-in-chief of a gynaecological journal, and the health magazine of *Der Spiegel*, she is the other co-founder of *Less — Doctors for Balance*.

OUR HORMONES, OUR HEALTH

how to understand your
hormones and transform
your life

Dr Susanne Esche-Belke &
Dr Suzann Kirschner-Brouns

Translated by Alexandra Roesch

SCRIBE
Melbourne • London

Scribe Publications
2 John St, Clerkenwell, London, WC1N 2ES, United Kingdom
18–20 Edward St, Brunswick, Victoria 3056, Australia
3754 Pleasant Ave, Suite 100, Minneapolis, Minnesota 55409, USA

Originally published in German as *Midlife-Care: Wie wir die Lebensmitte meistern und die Kraft unserer Hormone nutzen* by by Dr Susanne Esche-Belke and Dr Suzann Kirschner-Brouns

Published in English by Scribe 2021
Reprinted 2021

Printed and bound in the UK by CPI Group (UK) Ltd, Croydon CR0 4YY

Scribe is committed to the sustainable use of natural resources and the use of paper products made responsibly from those resources.

9781913348397 (UK edition)
9781950354719 (US edition)
9781922310224 (Australian edition)
9781925938753 (ebook)

Catalogue records for this book are available from the National Library of Australia and the British Library.

scribepublications.co.uk
scribepublications.com
scribepublications.com.au

Contents

Introduction

For some things in life there is a right time.

As doctors, mothers, wives, partners, friends, and hormone experts in our own right, we feel that now is the time.

Our midlife, with all its medical peculiarities, personal challenges and unforeseen opportunities, must be put into perspective at last. And that's what we'd like to do.

We hope this book helps to ensure that no woman over 40 has her symptoms dismissed by a doctor or is given inadequate treatment because, according to popular opinion, 'a woman who is still having periods can't be in menopause yet'. And, of course, we would like to play a part in ensuring that those who are in the midst of menopause and seeing a doctor for their symptoms feel taken care of in the best possible way.

Nowadays hormonal imbalances are increasingly appearing several years earlier than previously, and we consider this a neglected symptom complex. In this sense, *Our Hormones, Our Health* is the first book on treating menopause that deals with the hormonal changes that occur before menopause and puts these into context (thyroid, stress, gut, nutrition, sex hormones, and endocrine disrupters).

Let's be aware that we are the first generation to benefit from the findings of fledgling sciences such as epigenetics, stress medicine, microbial research, and nutrition science. Moreover, it is still early days for menopause research. That is why, in this book, we've compiled the latest scientific discoveries, as well as our practical experience with thousands of patients, interesting facts from conversations, interviews, and letters, and our own personal stories. At this point, we need all the information we can get. We also look into the attitudes, desires, and needs of those going through menopause: what is worth holding on to, what might 'loving letting go' actually look like, and what does being a menopausal woman today entail? Which goals and dreams do women still want to fulfil and how can we do it successfully?

In this book, we frequently refer to our subjects as women. We want to acknowledge the fact that biology does not dictate gender, and that menopause is in no way essential to womanhood, nor is it exclusive to the experiences of women. We want to extend our welcome to menopausal people who do not identify as women, and ask your forgiveness and patience as we navigate what is unfortunately very tricky territory within a patriarchal world. It is our sincerest hope that this work can be furthered and expanded on, and that one day soon, we might have access to books about trans and gender-nonconforming experiences of menopause, written by trans and gender-nonconforming authors. We have tried to reach a linguistic compromise by using gender-neutral and binary language interchangeably throughout this book. We hope that your reading experience is an empowering one.

We want to help you activate your inner doctor, so you can help yourselves, your children, friends, and colleagues get through this period of hormonal imbalance in a healthy and stable way.

With this in mind, we wish you a pain-free, energetic, stress-free, fulfilling, balanced, beautiful, exciting, sexy, and happy life.

1

The Hormonal Vortex

**Everything was fine, but all of
a sudden you don't recognise yourself?
We know that feeling all too well!**

The years of hormonal change are like a roller-coaster ride. They are
exciting and stressful at the same time. They are marked by extreme
ups and downs. Between those ups and downs, you survive one or
two loops on the ride. Your mood can escalate quickly from tense, to
nervous, to apprehensive. Your heart races, you start to sweat, you
get out of breath. Once you're back on firm ground, you might feel
pride mixed with wistfulness — pride because you survived the ride
and wistfulness that it's over. Change is a sign of life, whether that
change is thrilling and enriching, or scary and bewildering.

In the wise words of Danish philosopher Søren Kierkegaard,
'Life must be lived forwards and understood backwards.' That's
exactly how it was for us. We knew a lot about our bodies, but this
was always only in hindsight. It's surprising, because as doctors
we should have at least known, from a medical perspective, a fair
bit about the 'women's phase' that was coming for us as we moved
towards our forties. After all, we did attend gynaecology lectures
at university and completed one or two placements in gynaecology

departments. So, we can't deny that we are familiar with the regulatory hormonal circuits of the menstrual cycle. We know exactly when one of the two important female sex hormones, oestrogen, drops and when the other, progesterone, rises. No one needs to tell us about how hormonal fluctuations affect the body.

Or so we believed. We thought our study would prepare us for the hormonal fluctuations of menopause, and we could not have been more wrong! We had, of course, already felt the power of hormones in our own bodies, ever since adolescence. It's not an exaggeration to say that we have always experienced this strongly, both in the days before our period and shortly after childbirth. Did you proudly marvel at your growing breasts with the onset of puberty? And have you suffered from a tugging in your abdomen or mild-to-severe headaches in the days before your period? The former may have been due to a hormone boost and the latter to a hormone decline. The monthly hormone fluctuations associated with PMS (Premenstrual Syndrome) give 80 per cent of menstruating women abdominal pain, water retention, nausea, headaches, depressive moods, and many other symptoms. So, in this respect, things have been up and down for most women long before menopause.

Hormone fluctuations are particularly noticeable during pregnancy. The levels of oestrogen and progesterone are naturally very high for months. They ensure blood circulation in the pelvis and growth of the uterine lining, breasts, and placenta to care for the foetus. Hormone levels drop rapidly after birth. This results in almost all new mothers suffering from a depression between the second and tenth day after giving birth. Many new mothers are incredibly happy, and yet they experience waves of tears in those early days. As mothers, this is something we've both been through.

Suzann Kirschner-Brouns (SKB): 'When my husband came to my bedside on the second or third day after the birth and looked at me, out of nowhere I started sobbing violently. It came from the depths of my body. The outburst took us both

completely by surprise. As the tears poured down my cheeks,
I realised that we're right to call this hormone decline the
"baby blues".

However, being familiar with the power of female hormones as a
girl and young woman is just a small taste of what may later become
a permanent companion for several years: mental and physical
exhaustion, abysmal fatigue, feeling sad for no reason, depressive
mood disorders, malaise, headaches, and phases in which you're
almost manically happy or affectionate, like a teenager in love. And
these are just *some* of the symptoms of menopause.

Wait a minute, menopause? In your early or mid-forties? This is
a joke, right?

Not at all. See, the big mistake lies in misjudging the period of
time that menopause can have an effect. Hormonal changes and
corresponding symptoms can happen even when women are still
having periods. The fact that menopause does not start at the age
of 50 was confirmed by a study published in 2017 in the medical
journal, *Reproduction*. The study was conducted by Professor Gita
Mishra, Head of the Department of Epidemiology and Biostatistics
at the University of Queensland, Australia, and Director of the
Australian Longitudinal Study of Women's Health. The evaluation
of data from more than 51,000 women from Europe, Asia, and
Australia shows: if girls have their first period at a young age (under
11), then their risk of experiencing symptoms of hormonal imbalance
before the age of 44 is 80 per cent. If they have their first period at
the age of 12, then this risk is 12 per cent (at 13 years the risk is 9 per
cent). Moreover, women without children have double the risk of
an early menopause (in their early to mid-forties).

Symptoms caused by hormonal changes are recognised and treated
much too late in many women. Although there are medical clas-
sifications of premature menopause (before the age of 40), perimenopause (the onset of hormonal change until menopause), and

5

postmenopause (generally, 51+), in our minds — and this is the case for patients as well as therapists and doctors — there is an unshakeable notion that menopause relates exclusively to women over the age of 50. This is considered to be the age at which hot flushes and, in particular, other less obvious symptoms connected to changing hormone levels move into focus. It follows that it's only then that they are taken seriously and treated. In the first half of your forties, changing hormone levels are rarely acknowledged.

Even we as doctors — and the colleagues who treated us — didn't think very differently. This is why, in our early to mid-forties, we started running from pillar to post: to the orthopaedic surgeon because of newly occurring back and joint pain; to the neurologist because of sudden vertigo and migraine; to the cardiologist because of palpitations. We went to the dermatologist because of our sensitive skin and first-time allergies. And, of course, to the gynaecologist because of the sweaty, sleepless nights, the hair loss, the dry skin and the lack of libido. We looked at the kilograms that had settled almost overnight on our stomachs and hips just as dumbfoundedly as we sometimes looked at our colleagues, neighbours, and children — and our partners: 'Who are you? What do you want from us? Please just leave us alone!'

If we couldn't remember a name, or if we couldn't concentrate on anything anymore, we thought it was early-onset Alzheimer's. Those around us, and increasingly we ourselves, started to think we were hypochondriacs, or experiencing mental illness. And if all this wasn't already challenging enough, a depressive mood came along, which was truly gloomy and sometimes deeply sad. It robbed us of the last bit of strength.

Susanne Esche-Belke (SEB): 'I myself would have given a great deal for an expert colleague to have taken the time to explain the hormonal connections and show me a way out of the disaster zone. Then I would have known that hormonal changes don't start with menopause, i.e., when your periods stop at around the age of 51, but much earlier. Then I would have understood that my thyroid was applying the emergency brake, that my double burden as mother and doctor was weakening my adrenal glands, and that a glass of wine in the evenings was amplifying my oestrogen dominance. I would at least have been warned that in this phase of life, less would have been more. Instead there was too much of everything: too much oestrogen and cortisol in the blood, too much stress, too high an aspiration in the job and at home, wanting to make everything perfect. There was too much pressure, from myself as well, and I also still wanted to look good while all this was happening, despite one or two more pounds on my hips. But this came at the cost of my sleep.'

Like so many other people experiencing menopause, we were both hit hard. Suddenly (or perhaps sneakily), in the midst of life, our physical and mental confusion dictated our daily experience and wreaked chaos. We knew only this: we wanted our bodies back, we wanted to be able to think clearly again, we wanted to get on top of our moods again, we wanted to be pain free again and enjoy life. And apart from that — please, please let EVERYTHING be as it was before!

SKB : 'When I asked the gynaecologist whether hormones might be to blame, she replied: "Very unlikely — you're too young for that. We can do a test, but it won't tell us much. And if it were the case, then I wouldn't recommend hormone therapy — it's much too dangerous. You will have to get through this phase. That's the way it is, it's part of getting older."

"And how long will it last?"

"My dear colleague, it's not called the 'change of life' for nothing."

'I can still remember the bright-blue spring day and the blooming lilac in front of the gynaecologist's office in Munich. I barely made it down the stairs out into the street before the tears welled up. My nerves were shattered. I had two hours until the family got home, so I went straight to bed, pulled the covers over my head, switched my phone off, and hoped my child wouldn't need me. See no one, hear no one. I would worry another time about the article that I hadn't finished yet but needed to send to the editors by the next morning. Just not now.'

SEB: 'Although I've been a doctor for more than twenty years, have studied in five different countries, have worked in all departments, from emergency to intensive care, and have, alongside various professional developments, even completed a course in mindfulness-based stress reduction, I stumbled into the hormone chaos completely unprepared. It brought me closer to the edge than anything I'd experienced as a registrar, which I'd managed "easily" alongside running the home and bringing up three small children.

'In retrospect, of course, I ask myself how it could have happened: how did I slip into this phase so conspicuously — and yet undetected by myself and also by the colleagues I consulted about my symptoms? I was absolutely at a loss as to what was suddenly happening to me — a doctor and mother in the middle of my busy life. The fact was: my mental and physical state meant I could no longer manage my everyday life.'

SKB: 'After visiting the gynaecologist in Munich, I contacted two more colleagues. No one made a connection between my condition and perimenopause. I thought that after moving house several times, and having gone through a divorce, my personal circumstances had simply cost me too much strength, and that was why I was exhausted all the time. However, this was a new level of tiredness. It wasn't just my muscles that were exhausted, it was every single cell. My head felt weak, like I had a hangover, and my joints ached so badly some days that I was only able to drag my way through the day with the help of pills. When I took the dog for a walk around the lake, I needed three times as long for the return trip, which wound uphill through the forest. I was out of breath, my legs gave way, I had to rest several times on fallen tree trunks. Then I felt strong again for weeks on end and was as lively as a wild colt. Shortly afterwards, I lay on a mattress in the attic, stared at the bat nests, and listened to whale music the entire day. For weeks! Work, family, and my marriage all headed south.'

We knew alarmingly little about this phase of life. And ever since, we have noticed how few patients, readers, friends, and other women we meet know about their own bodies and their needs. As we said, professional help often isn't offered at the right time, because menopausal symptoms are either considered to happen several years later or dismissed as natural ageing processes. We're told that's just the way it is: your strength dwindles, your hair falls out, your muscles weaken. Pain? Who doesn't have some pain when they get older? Welcome to the club. Mothers pass on differing amounts and different kinds of 'women's business' to their daughters from culture to culture, and from family to family. Western cultures tend not to pass on much information to their daughters. In Western culture, we're taught not to talk about intimate things. Within families and even among friends, the prevailing belief is: 'I had to go through this by myself, so she'll manage somehow.'

We would like to oppose this with a firm No. In actual fact, we'd like to shout it out: NO! No woman has to 'manage' alone. After all, we no longer live in the 19th or 20th century, when many of the functions of the human body were still unexplored. Teeth are not pulled without local anaesthetic. Newborn babies are no longer operated on under anaesthetic but without pain relief, like they were until the 1980s. Until then, it was assumed that a newborn baby's nervous system was not developed enough to feel pain. Menopausal women no longer routinely have their uterus removed (known as a hysterectomy), as was happening well into the noughties, even when there was no real medical need for it. Until then it was assumed that after childbirth, the uterus was just a useless nuisance. And if the uterus was coming out, then you might as well remove the ovaries too. After all, what woman needs ovaries after the age of 50? According to a fact check carried out by the Bertelsmann Stiftung, in 2012 every sixth woman in Germany between the age of 18 and 79 no longer had a uterus. Predictably, male gynaecologists have proven to be quicker to pick up a scalpel than their female colleagues. Today we know how important the ovaries are for producing hormones — even after a hysterectomy. Who's surprised?

These days, such stories seem almost scandalous and 'medieval', but there are countless other examples that medicine, like any other social, political, and cultural field, underlies current levels of knowledge and research. In addition, there is the self-perception of the gender shift over time.

So, an even more emphatic *NO*.

Today we live in a historically unique situation. Triggered by protests in many countries across the world regarding abortion laws (the US, Ireland, and Germany, to name a few) and, most recently, by the impact of the #MeToo debate, many of us are finally experiencing self-determination over our bodies as well as real opportunities to stand up for ourselves and our needs. Women in their mid-forties are speaking up: they do not want to disappear into oblivion, along with everything they are and everything they have to offer. They can be competent, knowledgeable, and attractive, and they may be contributing to the economy and bringing up children and grandchildren, as well as being socially and politically active. All this doesn't suddenly stop just because a few hormones change. This issue has now been given a greater platform in respected publications. In the 24 June 2019 issue of *The New Yorker*, in a long opinion piece, American Harvard graduate and writer Sarah Manguso took a stance on the importance of the societal, social, and market-based power of menopausal women— a power that comes of liberation from being valued according to our looks and our fertility.

In Chapter 3, we will examine in detail the current state of studies on female hormones and will also address the different approaches to the topic of hormone replacement. But at this point we can say: the medical world is currently reconsidering the role of patients and is giving us a stronger voice in the decision-making process when it comes to our treatment.

There's another reason the time is right for a rethink: the average life expectancy for women 100 years ago was 52.5, partly due to the high maternal mortality rate during childbirth. This meant that at the beginning of the last century, far fewer women lived long enough to experience menopause. Since then, life expectancy has risen by almost 30 years, to an average of 83. So today we can indeed look gratefully and humbly at the years we probably have ahead of us.

Let's savour that once more: in the history of humanity, we are in an exceptional situation — we, in our forties and fifties, can ask the question of how we want to shape and spend the years to come. Many of us long for good health and, yes, being free from pain or chronic illness is a great asset in this long and important phase of life. At the very least, there are wonderful modern treatment options for hormone imbalances, so that symptoms caused by these can be mitigated very effectively.

We have excellent social opportunities and medical options to make these years happy, healthy, content, and active ones, in which we can pursue our projects and dreams. In every respect, we can go through hormonal change with new self-confidence. In countries with a public healthcare system, we have access to assistance in managing our health — namely, those long years of hormonal fluctuations. (In countries without public healthcare, access to this kind of support is still tenuous.) We have access to pioneering knowledge from epigenetics, stress medicine, nutritional medicine, and modern hormone replacement therapy in the form of bioidentical hormones. You don't need to struggle or suffer through it, and there is no reason to bury your head in the sand or 'soldier on'.

We are convinced that women are able to influence menopausal symptoms more positively than medicine and society as a whole thought us capable of until now. In fact, it makes sense to address the topic in your late thirties and early forties and to get preventative help. Be smarter than us! Start now — not after you've been in the attic for months with the bats, or at your window watching the leaves sailing down from the trees. And especially if you already find yourself 'in the thick of it', because even then, there are lots of things you can do to improve your physical and mental wellbeing.

It's essential that you don't regard (or treat) your body like a disappointing lover who has suddenly abandoned you, but as a good friend who has temporarily run into some difficulties. With knowledge, understanding, attention, and goodwill, you can find out what is wrong and what you need — for example, a well-tolerated therapy, bioidentical hormones, minerals, vitamins, and measures to reduce stress.

Another interesting aspect: it is said that the years between 40 and 50 are the time when your soul wants to grow. In other words, it is an important time for self-discovery. *Who am I, who do I want to be, what is important to me, and what is my task here on earth?* Some women report that it is only now that they experience a long sought-after 'return to self'. Urgent tasks required you to function externally, such as driving your career forward, starting a family, and building security for the future. You took on adult roles and had to do justice to them: the roles of parent, partner, adult daughter, or colleague. Now is a time when we might take stock and ask ourselves, *Who am I (still) behind all these roles?*

This is why we talk of self-care, self-compassion, and self-realisation. This sounds very selfish at first, but believe us, these topics have more to do with stress reduction and health than you might think.

Women continue to know very little about hormones and their effects on their body, energy, mood, performance, health, or weight. However, it is a fact that knowledge can provide tremendous motivation when it comes to health issues. If you understand why one measure makes sense and why the other is just a waste of money, then you can undertake a treatment or lifestyle change more consistently and easily. It's much easier to commit to doing something when it makes sense!

If you manage to integrate just a part of this into your daily life, you'll have a far greater chance of experiencing empowered, healthy, happy years ahead, free from the roller-coaster ride of hot flushes, migraines, osteoporosis, and mood swings.

We hope this book can provide clarity among the infinite, somewhat conflicting information that is currently available on the subject of hormones. To cover all facets and needs, it's important to bridge the gap between the different disciplines of conventional and non-conventional medicine; to incorporate psychology as well as other healthcare systems, such as traditional Chinese medicine, and to understand the links between body, mind, and medicine in restoring hormone balance.

As so-called evidence-based medicine, conventional medicine is based on the proven cause–effect principle. Various study designs, like the random distribution of study participants in what is known as a randomised double-blind trial, where neither the patient nor the doctor knows which drug is being used, are objective — you could even say, forgery-proof — and possess a correspondingly high reputation within science. Therapies that did not go through such a complex study procedure are not approved and often not paid for by health-insurance companies. This is the right approach in the case of drugs that have a strong effect on the body or mind and in the case of high-tech therapies. As trained medical practitioners who have ourselves carried out randomised studies, we fully support this.

That said, from our many years as doctors and medical journalists, we know that even in evidence-based medicine the situation is not always objective. Economic interests, lobbyism, and multiple other factors promote or guide the development of certain drugs or therapies, or prevent them. A lot of drugs are predominantly tested on healthy young men and not on women and children. This is why dosages or side effects for women often deviate from standardised recommendations. In addition, it has often been the case, in the history of pharmacology, that shortly after its release, a drug is praised to the skies, only to then be restricted or even banned because of 'unforeseen' side effects. For example, until 1977, Diethylstilbestrol (DES) was prescribed to hundreds of thousands of women in early pregnancy to prevent miscarriage. Later it was discovered that DES could cause damage to the foetus and increased the risk of vaginal cancer in daughters. There are also examples of the opposite: it used to be contraindicated to administer beta-blockers, a drug that lowers the heart rate, following a heart attack. Today it would be malpractice *not* to prescribe them.

We also know that compounds whose effect cannot be proven by exact studies are considered worthless. Up until a few years ago, doctors who claimed that the progression of chronic inflammatory bowel diseases (IBD) such as Crohn's disease and ulcerative colitis could be positively influenced by the administration of living bacterial strains, so-called probiotics, as well as bacteria-friendly nutrition with fermented foods, were considered by experts to be alternative. As the mechanism couldn't be proven by a randomised double-blind study, the mitigating effect on the illness, which could be observed in thousands of patients, was dismissed as a placebo effect or, even worse, as nonsense. That is, until the year 2001, when a newly developed technology deciphered all the genes in the human body and turned science upside down again. It was a sensation! Scientists later used this technology to identify the entirety of bacterial genes in a human body. By 2014, the time had come: it was determined that more than 100 trillion 'good' bacteria lived in the intestines, which not only strengthen our immune system and protect against infection, cancer, and much more, but also influence brain function. The knowledge that has been around for thousands of years, all over the world, about how important intestinal flora is for our health, and that these living bacteria can be specifically 'fed', has only been considered proven for six years now! Today no doctor would dare to denigrate a colleague who prescribed a probiotic to his patient, for example, to rebuild the intestinal flora after a course of antibiotics or to alleviate the symptoms of inflammatory bowel disease. This is just one example that demonstrates how reluctant we should be to condemn curative measures just because the relevant technical or biochemical detection method has not (yet) been discovered.

We are therefore presenting you with the latest evidence-based studies from varying disciplines, as well as guidelines and examples from medical practice, including valuable medical insider tips. But we are also going to introduce measures that are yet to undergo that stringent testing process, but which have provided many women with symptomatic relief, or had a preventative effect. This book was originally written for a German audience, and contained references to German statistics and studies. Where possible, we have updated these for English-language readers, but we urge you to check with the health-care providers in your own country for the most up-to-date recommendations. We've also included some resources for Australia, the UK, and the US at the end.

Midlife care starts now

'Middle age' is defined as the years between 40 and 55. Statistically speaking, most women go through their last menstrual cycle around the age of 51. According to the definition, menopause begins one year after the last period (so a 'pause' from menstruation is not entirely accurate. Meno*end* would be more correct). At this point, the lucky ones who don't suffer from menopausal symptoms now experience hormonal change, resulting in an end to their periods.

As previously mentioned, it is not always the case that women begin to experience hormonal changes in their late forties — often, this begins five to ten years earlier. Many women in their early forties notice that their bodies and/or their mental states are changing. And during life's rush hour, of all times! You may have started a family, or moved to a new city or into a new home; you may be getting established in your career, expanding your circle of friends, taking care of your parents, looking after your appearance, and dealing with myriad other things. No wonder that you get exhausted more often and more quickly than before. Your libido diminishes, your trousers feel tight, and it feels like a general heaviness weighs down on your life. When in actual fact, life has become rich and full! You could be really proud of yourself. Pause and pat yourself on the back — in many situations, that would be a good thing to do, perhaps even the only sensible option. Instead, your nerves grow ever more frayed.

This state of affairs doesn't imply a lack of willpower or organisational skills, diminishing ambition, or failure as mothers or partners. Very likely it is because the hormone levels are doing their own thing and this leads to specific symptoms, accompanied by irritating feelings. Who did this body used to be? Can it ever be trusted again?

'I have no idea what's wrong with me. I am just not myself anymore.' Maybe this sentence seems familiar because your muscles are aching again, or you can't get out of bed in the mornings because you feel too weak. Or maybe it's because at the most inconvenient moments, you feel completely deflated. It may not seem much consolation right now, but two-thirds of all women between the ages of 40 and 60 suffer from slight-to-severe menopausal symptoms — only a third remain symptom-free. Mood swings, emotional instability, weepiness, 'nerves' — there are lots of ways to describe this sudden state, where nothing is as it was before. The questionnaire in Chapter 3 will help you find out where you stand right now. Because the symptoms can also be caused by additional hormonal imbalances, such as hypothyroidism or adrenal fatigue as a result of chronic stress, we will also be examining these hormones.

> SKB: 'Fortunately, I never lost my composure at work, but I certainly did more than once in other situations. I remember a dinner in a restaurant when I suddenly started to cry. I couldn't calm myself down, so I eventually got up and fled to the toilets while the other guest looked on sympathetically. They probably thought I had argued with my friends or something like that, but it wasn't the case at all. It had actually been a joyful occasion: an acquaintance had given a friend's son as a school-leaving gift an old gold coin, which they had brought with them when they fled from Iran. They weren't my friends and the boy wasn't my son, and yet I was so moved by it that it took me 20 minutes to compose myself and return to the table. In other moments, a single word from my son or my mother could put me in a similar situation. I am totally fine with showing emotion, and I'm not embarrassed by a few tears, but it is a very strange feeling when a single word or gesture can leave you feeling overwhelmed by your emotions.'

The list that follows shows some of the possible symptoms and, believe us, we have had to go through quite a few of them ourselves.

And the few things we didn't experience personally have been passed on to us firsthand — from patients and friends, in interviews and in conversations that we have had in our professional and private lives.

SYMPTOMS THAT CAN OCCUR DURING PERIMENOPAUSE

Physical symptoms

- Hot flushes
- Loss of energy
- Dry eyes (contact lenses are more difficult to tolerate)
- Vague muscle and joint pain
- Headaches/migraines
- Severe PMT
- Loss of concentration, forgetfulness
- Nervousness
- Hair loss
- Weight gain
- Insomnia
- Decreasing libido
- Vaginal dryness
- Pain during intercourse
- Increase in allergies and asthma

Psychological symptoms

- Mood swings (more prone to crying, easily irritated)
- Melancholia and depressive moods (feeling empty, sad, emotionless, joyless)
- Anxieties
- No desire for sex
- Feeling burned out to the point of total exhaustion
- Brain fog (fuzzy feeling in the brain, feeling dizzy, foggy)
- No longer seeking a challenge, feeling curious, or having ambitions or goals

- Lack of energy to achieve any goals
- Reduced resistance to stress
- Drop in performance (less resilience)
- Inner anger (with permanent muscle tension, teeth grinding at night)
- Relationship issues

There is no script to address all these symptoms — like people, they are all individual. One patient might only have physical symptoms, like hot flushes and vaginal dryness, while another might have mood swings and brain fog. Many changes occur from one day to the next. You can also get a combination of symptoms. For example, you may be less able to concentrate, and if you then don't finish your work or do it properly, you might experience increased stress. As a result, your nerves may well be shattered. Or you wake up soaked in sweat and have to change your sheets or your pyjamas several times a night. No wonder your sleep pattern gets disrupted. Lack of sleep or poor sleep burdens the immune system, making you more prone to infections.

So, you quickly end up fighting on quite a few fronts. How, then, are you supposed to have an overview — especially if, from one second to the next, mundane things suddenly blow up in front of you, so that you feel like you are facing Mount Everest? You stand there and blink in disbelief and despair at the obstacle that yesterday was just an innocent shopping list, a harmless telephone conversation, or a plant that needs water. *Rien ne va plus* — nothing works anymore. At least, not as calmly and happily or contentedly as it used to, or as you would like it to. It can be really easy to allow harsh self-talk to enter the picture at moments like this. *Stop being so ridiculous, pull yourself together*, you think to yourself, half surprised, half annoyed — and you might hear your nearest and dearest say the same thing to you, too.

If at this point you can't find help from doctors, if neither the spa weekend nor the holiday leads to lasting relaxation, and if every morning the day is already over at 6.30 am because your child has slammed the bathroom door in your face, making you feel as bad as if your cat had just died — then this is the time when the mind games start: *Do I have a rare chronic disease that no doctor can diagnose? Can I no longer do my job properly because I am such a mess? Am I suffering from burnout? Am I going mad?*

No, we can reassure you, you are not going mad — this is all completely 'normal'. We emphasise that we only use the word 'normal' here to denote cause and effect, which means that a lack of oestrogen can make you feel weak and oestrogen dominance can make you feel restless and nervous. 'Normal' does not mean that you have to come to terms with this, for better or worse.

It is not a matter of tricking your biological clock into thinking that 50 is the new 30. We don't want to jump on the bandwagon of obsession with youth. This is a pointless battle that also leads to endless stress. Life means change; growing old can be nice; the first laughter lines around your eyes are a sign of a lot of joy and pleasure in life; a few kilograms more on the hips can look attractive. You can dye grey hair if you like. But those who desperately want to look 30 at 50, or feel the need to do so, are going along with a distorted image of women based on external, supposedly youthful beauty. We don't want to be part of that.

Instead, we want to support everyone in this phase of life to be able to go through these years healthily and harmoniously — physically and mentally — despite the hormonal changes. The emphasis here is on *healthy, vital, balanced, beautiful, and peaceful* — this goal should be 'normal' for all of us.

Case study: Depression or perimenopause

Anna was a 38-year-old scientist, married with no children. She came to see me in my surgery with a range of symptoms: lack of motivation, disrupted sleep, night sweats, irregular menstrual cycle, loss of libido, concentration issues in her demanding job, anxiety, and depression. Her professional life and her relationship were suffering the consequences, so Anna had been having psychiatric treatment and taking antidepressants. Yet despite the treatment, she still felt awful.

I thought she might be experiencing premature menopause. The psychiatrist regarded my suspicion as nonsense because Anna 'was still so young', and it took some time to dispel the scepticism. Finally, Anna agreed to let us test her hormone status.

The laboratory results confirmed my suspicion: her progesterone levels were barely detectable and her oestrogen levels were far below what they should have been.

We began an interdisciplinary, holistic therapy. The gynaecologist prescribed Anna bioidentical hormones (an oestrogen cream and pro-gesterone capsules) and a low dosage of DHEA (the main precursor of sexual hormones, the so-called 'Fountain of Youth hormone'). In addition, Anna was given a vitamin D supplement, and she reduced the sugar content of her diet. In consultation with her psychiatrist, the dose of her antidepressant was slowly reduced to zero. Anna continued to work on her anxiety and depression in her sessions with the psychiatrist.

Anna's condition stabilised from week to week. With the help of reg-ular doses of progesterone in the evenings, her sleep and concentration improved significantly. Her anxiety subsided, and she became more contented and even-tempered.

Six months later, she had lost a lot of weight, her relationship was back on track, and she was able to take on a senior management posi-tion, which meant a great deal to her.

If your doctor says, 'You're still having periods, so we don't need to test your hormones; taking a blood sample is a complete waste of time,' don't let yourself be fobbed off. Perimenopausal symptoms are real and they have to be taken seriously. Many health bodies advise hormone testing for women under 45 if they have the relevant symptoms.

SEB: 'As a general practitioner, for many years I have been treating patients with problems caused by physical and emotional instability. I have come to realise that many women unwittingly end up getting themselves into a state of emotional exhaustion during the years of perimenopause. Or they get no help because the classical laboratory results are "as expected", that is, within the normal range. It is worth taking a closer look here, as one patient may be feeling fine when her values are just within the normal range, while another may not. The spectrum can be very broad in terms of the values that are considered normal. So, a patient with latent hypothyroidism whose TSH value is still considered to be at the top end of the standard level might feel depressed and struggle to get out of bed, while another with the same values might be feeling completely fine. In my experience, the psychological impact often does not correspond to the laboratory results. This is why it is important that the therapy is not based solely on a number on a piece of paper, but also, and most importantly, on the patient's clinical condition.'

The relationship between doctor or therapist and patient is crucial. We seek relationships shaped by empathy and respect. However, the way modern medicine is practised can mean there may not be much opportunity for doctors to discuss patients' individual situations in detail or to discuss them with doctors in other disciplines. Doctors have to see a lot of patients in a short period of time, and there is too little time for 'talking medicine' — a conversation in a relaxed atmosphere that allows the patient to talk about themselves.

In no way do we want to call into question our colleagues and the many hard-working therapists who do a fantastic job with great dedication. We just wish there could more often be a broader approach that combines evidence-based conventional medicine, including classical laboratory medicine, with knowledge from naturopathy, psychology, and alternative therapies. This would allow the emotional and spiritual aspects of this phase of life to be better considered.

When professionals dismiss patients' symptoms, patients can return home from a medical appointment feeling frustrated and helpless (and don't forget that we doctors are also sometimes patients ourselves). This is exactly the experience we would like to spare you from going through. You should not be left alone with your problems. You should know what is going on in your body, what is the matter, and what might help.

KNOWLEDGE IS POWER

Information and knowledge are key to the reclamation of our bodies and our power. Fortunately, this is becoming increasingly available to many women around the world. For us here in Germany, 2019 marked the centenary of women's right to vote, and naturally, this sparked much writing about women's changing role in society. Today we are free to make decisions about our education, our choice of job, and our way of life. We are free to follow our dreams and no longer need to fight as a matter of principle for the right to study medicine, for example (as was the case in Germany until 1900), or to open our own bank account (as was the case until 1962), or to play football in a club (as until 1971). We now also legally control our own bodies. Even though there is still a lot to do on the equality front — for example in the matter of equal pay for equal work, women's prospects for career advancement, a partnership-based arrangement for raising children, medicines tailored to women's needs, and much more — we are relieved to be living in the year 2020.

Societal dictates still exist, but they are fading. Older, larger women are no longer described as 'matrons', you are less likely to hear snide comments in the changing rooms of fitness studios, and men are no longer getting laughs, even from their friends, when they make jokes like, 'The change of life is time to change your wife.' Even if these are stereotypical examples, and it may seem it's not worth even mentioning that we're leaving them behind, they at least show that we have moved on significantly.

Most of us can choose whether we want to start dyeing our hair or let it go grey, whether we want to look elegant in high heels or would rather walk comfortably in flats, whether our skirts end above or below the knee. We can have years of satisfying and experimental sex or we can crawl into bed with a book or a Netflix series. We can also have both: enjoy sex and then, for weeks afterwards, just enjoy time alone. To anyone who is reading this now and feeling pressure to go, as the saying goes, *higher, further, faster* – we'd like to say: you don't have to do anything. Be kind to yourself. We may be able to do more these days, and have lots of options open to us, but we don't need to prove anything.

There is also no shame in being at the mercy of your hormones. It has nothing to do with weakness. Nobody should be embarrassed to speak about their problems. And nobody with genuine symptoms should be sent away from a doctor's office having been labelled 'neurotic'.

This is exactly the feeling that many women have shared with us, even those who are otherwise happy with their lives. They report deeply humiliating situations in which they feel helpless and incapacitated, because they are not taken seriously by the medical profession. Don't shy away from tackling your problems – there are a lot of treatment solutions out there. And always remember: there are many people in the same situation as you!

SEB: 'The conversations with my patients over the last few years have given me a completely different view of my profession and of my life. I am infinitely grateful for the openness and the trust placed in me. I often notice that many colleagues completely disregard hormones when they are treating patients above the age of 35. Patients have told me that their doctors did not want to test their hormone levels, justifying this by saying that the values would change too often, that the health insurance companies would not cover the cost, or that they were still having periods, implying that there could not be a hormonal disorder. But with so many symptoms that I encounter in my daily practice, hormones *have* to be factored in as a cause within the treatment strategy. For example, so many women in their mid-thirties have been suffering from undiagnosed thyroid dysfunction. These women are often only diagnosed when they need help getting pregnant.'

How hormones steer our body and mind

One-millionth of a gram or even one-trillionth of a gram per litre of blood is often enough hormone to produce a reaction. This can also happen really fast: when you get upset or are in a stressful situation, the hormones adrenaline and noradrenaline will kick in at the drop of a hat. Other hormones, like the thyroid hormone, take days to have an effect.

Adrenaline was the first hormone to be isolated in 1895. Since then, around 150 different hormones have been discovered in our bodies. However, it is estimated that there are well over a thousand. They are primarily produced in the six large hormonal glands: the hypothalamus, pituitary gland, thyroid, pancreas, adrenal glands, and male or female reproductive glands (gonads). Additionally — this is something a lot of people don't know — smaller quantities of hormones are produced in other body tissues, such as fatty tissue, blood, and the intestine. They reach their target cells via the blood, stick themselves like a key into a matching keyhole, the receptor, and set the relevant effect in motion.

At the top of the list are the hypothalamus and the pituitary gland, both endocrine glands in the brain. They secrete hormones that regulate other hormonal glands. For example, thyrotropin-releasing hormone (TRH) steers the release of hormones from the thyroid and follicle stimulating hormone (FSH) stimulates hormone production in the ovaries and testicles.

Some hormones are antagonists, such as insulin and glucagon. This means that their effects are mutually dependent. The former lowers the blood sugar and the latter raises it, so that in an ideal situation, the blood-sugar levels are balanced. Other hormones act like dominoes: TRH from the hypothalamus stimulates the pituitary gland to release thyroid-stimulating hormone, and this in turn causes the production of thyroid hormones in the thyroid gland. Hormones such as oestrogen and progesterone work together — in pregnancy, both cause the endometrium of the uterus to grow.

The hormonal cycle is determined by supply and demand, or rather, shortage and replenishment. Because the tiniest amount of a single hormone can have such an impact and because hormonal control loops are so complex, the system is quite vulnerable to stress and sleep deprivation, among other things. Anyone who has ever experienced jet lag can tell you a thing or two about what it feels like when the sleep hormone, melatonin, is out of sync.

We will be examining the most important hormones and their cycles more closely in Chapter 2. There you can read everything about the skin and hair hormone oestradiol and the many miracles it can perform. We will also be looking at the bonding hormone, oxytocin, the stress hormone cortisol, and those hormones that bring us *to take action,* as well as those that are responsible for mild hunger pangs or that have an appetite-suppressing effect.

HORMONES DETERMINE OUR SEXUAL CHARACTERISTICS

Oestrogen and progesterone are *the* ultimate female hormones. They cause breasts to grow in puberty and the hips to round; they control menstruation and make pregnancy possible. But they also ensure smooth skin and strong hair. The splendid long hair that a lot of young girls have is a good demonstration of this: thanks to oestrogen, their hair is healthy and shiny. However, there is not one single oestrogen, but a number of oestrogens that form an entire group of more than 30 female sexual hormones. (Note: It's common practice to speak of oestrogen rather than oestrogens; we will use both interchangeably throughout this book, depending on the context.) Oestrogen controls the female cycle, increases blood circulation in the uterus, promotes the storage of fluid in tissues, affects bone density, and has a positive effect on blood lipids. Progesterone also regulates menstruation and pregnancy by protecting the mucous membrane of the uterus and helping to stabilise emotions.

The Head of Paediatric Endocrinology and Diabetology from University Hospital Ulm, Martin Wabitsch, is an expert in his field and, through his research, he has concluded that 'hormones are the key to our behaviour and personality'.

In this sense, the female hormones form not only our body, but also our character. We should be aware that through these hormones, especially oestrogen, we are more inclined to have nurturing qualities. Throughout history, this has ensured the survival of newborn babies, who might otherwise have starved to death. Nonetheless, we are of course very happy that more and more men are now involved in caring for their babies and children every day.

Oestrogen also ensures a cheerful disposition as well as emotional balance. But our character is not only shaped by the sex hormones — cis men possess more testosterone, cis women more oestrogens — but also by the other players in our bodies. If more cortisol is produced naturally, for example, then a person is probably more stressed and aggressive. If there is more oxytocin present, then this person is probably more loving and emotionally balanced.

Interestingly, the beginning of the hormone roller-coaster often coincides with the time when women are starting to feel that they have had enough of their role as carers within a family, in social communities, or at work. We recently overheard a woman at the next table in a café saying, 'I'm so tired of worrying about everyone and taking care of them.'

If you are feeling the same way, this might also have something to do with your evolutionary 'provider hormone', oestrogen, reducing. But don't feel guilty about it — nature is pretty clever. It knows that now is the time to no longer pass on your energy to everyone else, but rather to use some of it for yourself. Female testosterone, which is responsible for this change in motivation, is not going to be reducing for a long time yet.

What do you need to make you feel good? (This is a question that we will be asking you often in this book.) Who would you like to be? Where do you want to be in life? What do you want to experience? How do you want to feel in the many fantastic years to come?

2

The Hormone Carousel

Before we introduce you to the alchemy of female hormones and consider the question of *what* hormones actually are, we first want to give a sense of their nature, examining *how* they do what they do. So, we'd like you to do some imagining for a moment:

Imagine a princess. This princess is very beautiful. She has long shiny hair and radiant, smooth skin. She is cheerful, kind, sensitive, even-tempered, caring, and alert. Her behaviour is purposeful. She manages challenging situations without ever losing her nerve. She seems to glow from within.

When both of us were growing up, we longed to be princesses. We idolised these celestial beings. But if we are completely honest, we probably also secretly wondered how princesses got to be so perfect. Just before falling asleep, we might have thought, *Something is not quite right here.*

The princess can't manage it all alone — there must be a huge crowd of invisible helpers working away behind the scenes. And it can't just be the seven dwarfs. There must be lots of them — thousands and thousands of invisible creatures, fairies, fairy godmothers, and magical animals.

They probably cater to her every whim, comb her hair, bathe her, treat her skin with precious oils, feed her and bring her drinks, encourage her to walk around the magic garden, and harness the horses to her golden carriage. And when the carriage stops in front of the castle after a delightful drive through the magic forest, the princess alights, beautiful and happy, and nimbly mounts the steps.

Yes, that's how it must be ...

Now, you might not be the princess type, but humour us for a moment here (and please excuse us if imagining your body as a princess is unappealing to you!). Imagine the whole body as the princess. Inside the body, thousands and thousands of invisible little helpers carry out miracles: these helpers are our hormones. At their best, which means when we have enough of them and in the right balance, they are the Fountain of Youth. This is true, even if the German Cancer Research Centre (DKFZ) warns against only using hormones in later life as 'wrinkle smoothers'. The fact is that hormones turn children into young adults.

Hormones stir us up

Hormones dictate our daily rhythm, stabilise our immune system, keep our brain fit, strengthen our bones, stimulate our digestion and blood circulation, and regulate our appetite and core body temperature. They steer muscle and bone growth, the menstrual cycle, our feelings, our moods, and countless other elements of our physical and mental experience.

The key to good hormonal health is balance. Too much or too little of a certain hormone can affect our health swiftly and dramatically. For example, thyroid hormone deficiency may result in weight gain, tiredness, and constipation; while an overproduction can cause weight loss, anxiety, and palpitations.

Endocrinology, the study of hormones, is a relatively new field of medicine. Ernest Starling was the first scientist to understand the significance of the endocrine, or hormone-producing, glands. Their existence had been described anatomically and the thyroid and adrenal glands had been identified, but no one really knew what they did. Thankfully, this is different today, but there is still a great deal to be explored in this field.

Hormones are primarily produced in the six large hormonal glands: the hypothalamus, pituitary gland, thyroid, pancreas, adrenal glands, and male or female reproductive glands (gonads). They deposit hormones into the circulating blood, which sometimes transports them to distant destinations: for example, from the pituitary gland to the ovaries, or from the thyroid down to the intestine. Once they arrive at the target organ or cell, they dock onto receptors and set the corresponding effect in motion. For example, adrenaline and noradrenaline kick in during stress, melatonin makes us sleepy, and ghrelin makes us hungry.

Alongside the endocrine glands, which distribute their hormones via the blood, there are exocrine glands that distribute them externally, for example, through the saliva, sweat, or mammary glands, using their secretion to deposit the hormones where they are needed.

Most hormones are team players and their reciprocal impact is extremely complex. From time to time, this hampers the diagnosis of a hormone-related disorder. If one of them is not performing properly, this can affect the others. In such a complex system, when something is awry, it can be very tricky to get to the root of the matter. Moreover, when you begin to track the hormones, their circuits and their effects, you often come to realise that a symptom has more than one cause.

This is why we will be introducing not only female hormones in this chapter, but also some other very important hormones. Of all the systems at work in our body, it is our hormones that work together most closely.

Let's begin our exploration.

The female sex hormones

Let's think back to that princess: do you have thick, shiny hair and smooth skin? Is your vagina moist with good blood circulation when you feel like sex? Do you even feel desire? Do you have a regular heartbeat with no signs of high blood pressure? Is the only time your muscles and joints ache the day after a half-marathon, or the first day of a hiking trip? Are you still having periods, with light symptoms of PMT, but otherwise you feel strong, well adjusted, and attractive? If you decided you wanted a baby, did you get pregnant straightaway, have an uncomplicated pregnancy, and the baby is doing just fine? If all that is the case, then it looks as though your oestrogen and progesterone levels are exactly as they should be.

Nonetheless, you are reading this book and we think this is very wise. To continue to feel well, it's worth finding out all there is to know about hormones before there is anything to worry about.

THE BRAIN: YOUR MENSTRUAL CYCLE BEGINS HERE

Most of us spend a lot of time strategically planning and imagining our future. We might lie awake at night thinking about which outfit to wear for a particular event, or what gift our partner might like for their anniversary, or when the right time might be to ask for a pay rise. We imagine using this pay rise and picture ourselves lying on a Caribbean beach or on a new sofa. We can also spend a whole lot of time worrying about our future — our financial stability, our physical health and strength, our relationship status, and so on. Lots of us also spend a lot of time mulling over our past; what-iffing, reliving, and grieving. And then there are the thousands of fleeting thoughts that we are not even aware of.

But our brain can do a lot more than just thinking and dreaming. It is the seat of the most important control centres of our hormone cycles: the hypothalamus and pituitary gland.

If you were to draw a horizontal line from the bridge of your nose towards the back of your head and a vertical line from the top of your head towards your neck, the hypothalamus would be right where those two lines meet. It secretes 'releasing hormones' that stimulate the production of hormones in other glands, which then release them into the bloodstream. This is how the hypothalamus controls things such as body temperature, heart rate, and blood pressure.

The hypophysis or pituitary gland is the size of a cherry stone and hangs directly beneath the hypothalamus. It controls the thyroid, the adrenal glands, and the ovaries (and thus, the menstrual cycle). To trigger the phases of the menstrual cycle, it produces the follicle-stimulating hormone (FSH), which causes the egg to ripen and increases oestrogen production, as well as the luteinising hormone (LH) for ovulation.

The hypothalamus and pituitary gland are powerful organs — they dictate most of the other hormonal glands' activity. Once the desired hormone concentration has been reached in the bloodstream — this is measured by a sort of thermostat or sensor — the brain receives negative feedback. The brain signals to the hormonal glands in the rest of the body, 'Pause, pending further notice.' Supply and demand — or rather, shortage and replenishment — dictate the hormonal cycles.

THE MENSTRUAL CYCLE

Every newborn girl comes into the world with more than a million egg cells. These are all the egg cells that she will ever have. It sounds like a lot and it is; however, we have to be economical with them. Later, from the first period onwards, the body draws on this pool, which consists of 'only' 300,000 to 400,000 eggs. During a woman's lifetime, approximately 500 of these egg cells will mature. This means that the egg cells of a 25-year-old woman are 25 years old, and those of a 40-year-old woman are 40 years old.

Maturing takes place in the ovaries in a small, pouch-like structure called a follicle. This contains the female egg cell and the oestrogen-forming cells. The more the follicle grows, the more oestrogen is released. Over the first 14 days of a cycle, this ensures the growth of the egg cell and also the uterine lining, so that an egg that is eventually fertilised can find a cosy, secure bed where it can lodge itself.

Around day 14, the follicle bursts, releasing the egg, which then travels through the fallopian tube to the uterus. During the second half of the cycle, the luteal phase, the follicle remains in the ovary and transforms into the corpus luteum, the 'yellow body' of the ovary. This gland now produces the corpus luteum hormone, progesterone. It ensures that the uterine lining continues to thicken and is better supplied with blood.

PHASES OF PERIMENOPAUSE
Hormonal changes take place in three phases

Phase one:
Perimenopause begins
with the decline of
progesterone levels

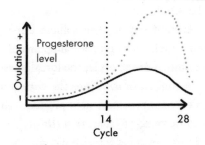

Phase two:
Later, oestrogen
levels also drop

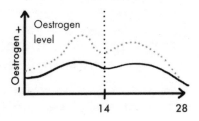

Phase three:
Postmenopause — now
the basal oestrogen
level also declines

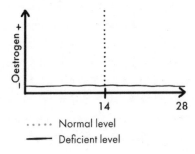

..... Normal level
—— Deficient level

If the egg is not fertilised, then the message, 'As you were!' is conveyed and the corpus luteum fades away. As a result, the concentration of progesterone and oestrogen drops. The uterine lining, which has received increased blood supply, is shed, as it is no longer required. This is menstruation.

> SEB: 'Our hormones have the power to determine our sexual characteristics. Objectively, they ensure the survival of humanity by controlling reproduction. I get very enthusiastic about this, but hormones are responsible for the miracle of life. Time and time again I find myself amazed that our sexual hormones enable a completely new, unique, living being to form from two cells. After all these years as a mother and doctor, this still fills me with humility and joy.'

HORMONES ARE THE SOURCE OF OUR PHYSICAL AND MENTAL WELLBEING

Oestrogen and progesterone belong to the group of steroid hormones. Cholesterol, which you probably know of as blood fat, provides the basic framework for these hormones. They are fat-soluble and can therefore zoom through cell membranes and enter the cell, as far as the cell nucleus. This makes them very efficient.

Oestrogen and progesterone have a profound influence on our body and our behaviour. Oestrogen affects our levels of happiness and our emotional equilibrium, and progesterone affects our cortisol levels and calms our nervous system. Remember, as Martin Wabitsch from the University Hospital Ulm says, hormones are the key to our behaviour and personality.

OESTROGEN (ESTROGEN)

Oestrogen holds a seat of immense power among hormones. When our oestrogen levels are in balance, they can make us look glowing and feel energetic, healthy, calm, and clear-headed. When they are off balance, then our nerves can feel utterly shredded. Moreover, imbalanced hormones can stimulate adverse cell-growth.

Oestrogens form a group of more than 30 messenger substances. As well as in the ovaries, they are produced in the fatty tissue, in small amounts in the testicles, and in a region of the brain that is important for learning and memory. In 2001, scientists from the Max Planck Institute of Psychiatry in Munich provided the biochemical proof that oestrogens act like neuroprotective antioxidants. They protect nerve cells and their connections (synapses) by intercepting aggressive and damaging molecules and proteins. In this way, they defend our brain in situ. (Maybe this is why we often know the answer to our partner's question: 'Darling, do you know where I left my car keys?')

The three most important endogenous oestrogens are oestradiol, oestrone, and oestriol. They cause the follicle to ripen, trigger ovulation, and ensure that the egg is transported through the fallopian tube to the uterus. They stimulate the growth of the uterine lining, breasts, and vaginal cells, as well as the secretion of mucus at the cervix. This cervical mucus acts as a natural barrier against external germs. Oestrogens also make our pubic hair grow.

However, the effect of oestrogens is not limited to the sexual organs. Within the rest of the body, they stimulate blood flow, strengthen the immune system, and stimulate the production of proteins, leading to an increase of triglycerides and cholesterol in the blood and water retention in the tissues. High oestrogen levels are linked to a higher risk of thrombosis and some types of cancer, and to depression and being overweight. Excess oestrogen can also lead to liver damage.

Unfortunately, all oestrogens are often lumped together and demonised as a cause of breast cancer in the context of oestrogen levelling during menopause. But this is far from the full story (we will explain more in Chapter 3).

Insights into the protective function of oestrogens have primarily been gleaned from research into menopause. In the words of Joni Mitchell: *You don't know what you've got till it's gone ...*

With this in mind, we would like to emphatically highlight the protective effect of oestrogen. Among other things, this concerns osteoporosis, a bone disease that affects 80 per cent of women during and after menopause. Because the ratio of bone build-up and bone loss is impaired, the bone becomes more porous and brittle. This can often result in the fracture of the femoral neck, but can also cause damage to other typical weak spots such as the pelvis, spine, and lower arm. According to a bone evaluation study on the epidemiology of osteoporosis, in Germany, one woman in four above the age of 50 as well as 1.1 million men are at risk. More than half of the patients who develop osteoporosis will suffer a broken bone within the space of four years, according to guidelines from the Wissenschaftlichen Dachverband Osteologie in 2017.

Oestrogens also protect against arteriosclerosis, cardiovascular disease, and Alzheimer's disease. From the age of 65, women are twice as likely to be diagnosed with Alzheimer's as men. New findings show that this illness particularly affects the hippocampus, an area of the brain where oestrogen production drops dramatically during menopause.

Oestrogens also lower our risk of getting certain types of cancer. The 2016 international guidelines for hormone replacement suggest that oestrogens can prevent bowel cancer. The risk of bowel cancer is halved after nine to 14 years of hormone replacement therapy. How does this work? Oestrogen receptors have anti-proliferative and anti-inflammatory effects; they can stop cell growth and inhibit inflammation. Oestrogens are not only used as preventative medicine, but are also therapeutically administered to bowel cancer and prostate cancer patients. In their current recommendations for preventing cancer, the German Cancer Society notes a reduced risk of breast cancer through oestrogens given via the skin during menopause.

Let's take a look at the most important natural oestrogens. Each plays a different role, and this becomes important when we start considering hormone replacement therapy.

OESTRADIOL (E2, BETA-OESTRADIOL, ESTRADIOL)

Oestradiol is a natural oestrogen that is formed in the ovaries and in the placenta. Men produce it in their testicles and adrenal cortex. It is the most effective and therefore most important oestrogen. As is the case for all sex hormones, the originating substance is cholesterol, which is why oestradiol is formed from body fat in the stomach, hips, and thighs. This is also why larger women tend to have a higher oestradiol level.

Oestradiol triggers ovulation and prepares the lining of the uterus for the implantation of a fertilised egg.

It is vital as protection against osteoporosis, ensures strong bones, helps prevent wrinkles and greasy skin, and strengthens our hair. This is why it is celebrated as the *skin and hair hormone* by the media. It makes our blood vessels elastic and protects against arteriosclerosis and high blood pressure. After menopause, the body's production of oestradiol falls and oestrone increases.

OESTRONE (ESTRONE) AND OESTRIOL (ESTRIOL)

Oestrone and oestriol are interchangeably converted into one another by the body, depending on food, liver function, alcohol, stress levels, and so on. Before menopause, oestrone plays a less important role and is produced at a lower rate. Production increases after menopause, which protect our bones — but because it stimulates cell division, it also promotes cancer.

Oestrone is produced almost equally in the ovaries and in the

41

subcutaneous fatty tissue, and to a lesser extent in the adrenal glands. In the subcutaneous fatty tissue, it is formed by androstenedione, a male hormone. Large menopausal women with strongly developed subcutaneous fatty tissue usually have a higher oestrone level. Higher levels of oestrone can be caused by regular consumption of alcohol, a fatty liver, and a genetically determined overactivity (CYP19 mutation) of the enzyme aromatase, which converts androstenedione to oestrone.

PROGESTERONE — BALM FOR THE NERVES

Progesterone is the second-most important female sex hormone. On the one hand, it complements the effect of oestrogen; on the other, it is its antagonist. The two are intimately related: progesterone balances out our oestrogens, and without oestrogen, progesterone cannot fully take effect. Together they determine the menstrual cycle. They make conception possible and allow an embryo to develop. It is immensely important to our wellbeing that these two hormones work well together.

Progesterone is produced in the follicle cell from cholesterol. After ovulation, the level of progesterone surges. With the help of progesterone, all the structures in the lining of the uterus (cells, blood vessels, glands, and so on) are changed and prepared for the implantation of the fertilised egg cell. This ensures that an embryo's needs are adequately supplied. Later in the pregnancy, huge amounts of progesterone are produced (up to 300 times the normal value) in the placenta. If pregnancy does not occur, the level of progesterone falls, and the prepared mucous membrane is discharged during menstruation.

Progesterone acts not only on the uterus but on almost all body tissues, in the brain as well as in the peripheral nerves. It is important for the immune system, energy production, temperature and water regulation, and bone and fat metabolism. It lowers the risk of various types of cancer and intensifies the effect of thyroid hormones.

Under the influence of progesterone, our body temperature increases by around 0.5 degrees during the second half of the cycle, on the days around ovulation. By monitoring this change in temperature, women can tell when they are ovulating. Natural contraception is based on this principle; there is even an app for it.

Together with oestrogen, progesterone guards against osteoporosis and encourages new bone growth. Its vital role in the maturation of the central nervous system is deeply underestimated. The concentration of progesterone is up to 20 times higher in certain brain cells than in the blood. A research group from the department of cytology at the Institute for Anatomy at Ruhr University Bochum is currently researching the question of whether progesterone can regenerate nerve cells in stroke patients.

Allopregnanolone in particular, which is formed in the brain and spinal cord, has a protective role in the central and peripheral nervous system. This is possibly why we are better able to concentrate and think when our progesterone level is high. As progesterone also docks onto the receptors for neurotransmitters (GABA receptors), it has a similar effect to the sedative diazepam (first marketed as Valium). Progesterone has a calming effect and helps us to sleep better. In this sense, progesterone also reduces stress.

Progesterone strengthens the immune system, and acts as an anti-inflammatory and also as a diuretic, flushing out fluids and therefore tightening connective tissue. It increases libido, especially around the time of ovulation.

This all-rounder is not exclusive to women; men also produce progesterone. It's crucial to the production of testosterone.

OXYTOCIN — ROSE-COLOURED GLASSES

First impressions count. We usually know immediately whether we like someone or not. Maybe we even get butterflies in our tummy. Our oxytocin levels are not entirely blameless here.

Even though it is not a sex hormone, we felt that oxytocin, which is formed in the pituitary gland, belongs in this sub-chapter. It is known as the 'cuddle hormone'; it bonds us emotionally to our loved ones, and it is produced during orgasm.

It is the hormone that triggers contractions during labour and delivery, as well as breast milk production after giving birth. Because of the high levels of oxytocin produced during breastfeeding, the mother's cortisol levels decrease. In this sense, oxytocin reduces anxiety and relieves stress. Thanks to the relaxing effect of oxytocin, some mothers often experience breastfeeding as a moment of calm and enjoyment, which in turn is enjoyable for their babies.

If prairie mice — which are by nature monogamous — are given an oxytocin-antagonist, in other words, a substance that works against oxytocin, then they have sex with other partners, in contrast to their usual behaviour. There's a saying among scientists: 'Mice tell lies' — in other words, testing on mice cannot be relied on because mice are not the same as humans. However, it's still assumed that oxytocin increases our tendency towards bonding behaviour. To put it another way, the higher your oxytocin level, the more likely you are to be faithful to a partner.

Skin contact and sex encourage the production of oxytocin, which is why it's known as the cuddle hormone. In interpersonal contact, oxytocin encourages trust as well as emotional competence, especially when you touch the other person's lower arm, place your hand on their shoulder, or greet them with a kiss on the cheek, for example. But the touch needs to last at least twenty seconds to have an effect.

However, outside couple relationships this appears to primarily apply to women. Men react more critically to another person when they are under the influence of oxytocin, as a Chinese research team showed. After being given a dose of oxytocin in the form of a nose spray, the women in the study developed more positive feelings towards others, while the men grew more critical.

TESTOSTERONE — WE ARE ALSO A LITTLE BIT MASCULINE

Women not only have female but also male sex hormones, namely, androgens. The most well-known androgen is testosterone. Other male hormones are androstenedione and dehydroepiandrosterone (DHEA).

Testosterone is formed in the ovaries and in the pituitary gland. It directly affects the female body, but it can also be converted into oestrogen.

Around the age of 50, the ovaries stop producing eggs; however, low amounts of male and female hormones continue to be produced. This is known as basal production.

Testosterone gives us assertiveness and authority. It affects our vitality and our libido. It is the driving force that makes many women in this phase of life want to shake their life up a bit. This often leaves partners perplexed. But testosterone can help you not give a damn.

DHEA is the most frequently formed hormone in the body. Alongside its function as a prohormone (a hormone that is not yet active) for sex hormones, it is also an antagonist for the stress hormone cortisol. It is considered the ultimate anti-ageing hormone: it has many positive effects on the cardiovascular system and the brain, and is a supporter to the mitochondria — the power plants in our cells. DHEA reduces fatty tissue and builds up muscles, regulates body weight, improves the immune defences, and makes you better able to deal with stress.

The concentration of DHEA is highest when we are in our twenties and thirties — after that, the level sinks continuously. This may be one of the reasons for the increased stress sensitivity and susceptibility to infections that we see with increasing age, and maybe for the ageing process itself. While the body (unfortunately) continues to produce the same amount of cortisol, its antagonist goes into retirement, so to speak. And now we have arrived at what often appears to be the ultimate villain — cortisol. But be careful with those preconceptions: there's more than one side to everything.

The stress hormones

Our stress behaviour is also steered by hormones. Triggered by a shock or as a reaction to a perceived threatening event, our heart races and our legs tremble. Those who have managed to survive a life-threatening situation know that our body's alarm system guarantees that we don't waste a single second reflecting. It incites us, so to speak, to jerk the wheel violently on the motorway to avoid the obstacle instead of asking ourselves: 'Do I want to run into the crash barrier?' That kind of reflection would be anything but productive. This is why we react in auto-pilot mode in situations like this.

But even when our minds are shut off, everything begins afresh in our heads. Our stress system functions across the hypothalamic-pituitary-adrenal axis (HPA axis). Watch out, here come a whole lot of hormone names: corticotropin-releasing hormone (CRH) and vasopressin are released from the hypothalamus, which cause adrenocorticotropin hormone (ACTH) to be released in the pituitary gland. This in turn activates the production and release of the stress hormones adrenaline and noradrenaline in the pituitary gland.

The adrenal glands are situated above the left and right kidney. If you place your hands on your waist with your thumbs facing forward and the other fingers on your back, then it is the spot where your little finger is. In very stressful moments, you can sometimes feel your adrenal glands pulsing.

Adrenaline and noradrenaline activate that part of the nervous system responsible for alertness — the sympathetic nervous system (SNS). The SNS, with its many branches, ensures that the organs that are indispensable during times of stress are adequately supplied with energy: heart, lungs, and muscles. As a result, the heart beats faster, blood pressure rises dramatically, and muscles tense and prepare to sprint away.

All humans respond to emergency situations with a fight, flight, freeze, or faun response. Gender plays a role in which response we're more likely to reach out for — men, in particular, tend to fight when attacked — but we're all capable of reacting in any of these four ways.

CORTISOL — THE OLYMPIC FLAME

Cortisol is produced in the adrenal cortex and is partially made from progesterone. It ensures that those bodily functions that are not urgently required for survival, like digestion, libido, or the immune defence (cold viruses will be taken care of later) are curbed. At the same time, cortisol also makes sure that the body maintains a low level of alertness. This costs energy, and therefore cortisol increases the release of insulin to mobilise sugar and triglycerides (fats) for the production of energy from the cells. Being alert isn't bad — many doctors say that a certain level of stress is needed to remain concentrated and resistant to infection.

But ...

As you might have guessed, if we are under persistent, chronic stress, then the adrenal cortex increases the production of cortisol, resulting in all organs being in a constant state of alertness. This is like keeping the accelerator in our car pressed to the floor, or constantly pulling all-nighters. In the long term this can lead to raised blood pressure, a rapid heartbeat, permanently tense and eventually tightly knotted muscles, a weakened immune system, constipation, decreased libido, and lower production of oestrogen, progesterone, and DHEA. The risk of osteoporosis and adrenal fatigue also increases.

The former happens because cortisol and progesterone compete for the same receptor at the bone cells. Progesterone helps with bone growth; high cortisol levels mean more manpower. The cortisol molecules displace the sex hormone at the receptor and the bones grow more brittle.

Chronic stress can lead to significant weight gain. Our brains in particular need more energy under stress. Even without stress, the human brain requires half of the carbohydrates we eat each day. This corresponds to approximately 14 tablespoons of sugar; in stressful times it easily needs up to 12 times that amount of 'nerve nourishment'. If you don't always have a bar of chocolate at the ready, then the brain uses up the sugar reserves that were intended for the muscles, organs, and cells, and these have to be replaced. The body demands an energy boost and demonstrates this through a decline in concentration, by making us feel queasy or causing our hands to shake. Hunger is stress, the alarm system revs up, cortisol levels increase, and we make a beeline to the fridge ...

HYPOTHALAMIC-PITUITARY-ADRENAL (HPA) STRESS AXIS

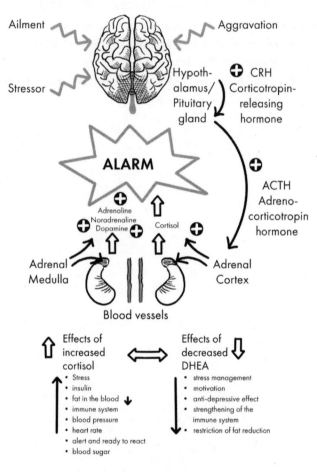

Some people lose weight when they are under a lot of stress. They grow thin because their brain takes energy from muscles and fatty tissue. In people who gain weight under stress, this mechanism does not work. They are forced to eat in order to feed their brain. In their case it would be a good idea to run three circuits around the office building after an argument with a colleague. But who's going to do that? This is why, in some people, the body likes to convert the extra non-metabolised energy into fat and store it around the stomach area.

The diagram on the opposite page demonstrates what happens when our systems undergo stress.

The metabolism hormones

INSULIN — THE MAGIC KEY

The hormone insulin stems from the pancreas. You can imagine it like a magic key without which the sugar derived from nourishment cannot reach the cells. It is needed for metabolic processes as the prime energy supplier. Insulin opens little 'doors' in the cells and carries in the sugar (glucose). But what happens if there is already enough sugar in the cells and they are full up? Well, then, Houston, we have a problem.

This is one explanation for 'the obesity crisis'. Many people eat more than their body needs in order to function well — especially sweets, ready-made meals with added sugar, and high-calorie products such as lemonade, alcohol, juices, and smoothies. Fruit contains fruit sugar, which is why pre-packaged smoothies in particular can contain more sugar than a glass of Coke.

This flood of sugar is a huge challenge for the pancreas. It has to produce enormous amounts of insulin to be able to clear the sugar from the blood in the cells. But the cells only put up with this for a certain amount of time. When what we eat on a daily basis is the kind of sugary food that should be reserved for sometimes, the body begins to reject this consistently high sugar intake in the only way it knows how. The cells protect themselves by locking their doors when sugar comes knocking. This state is called insulin resistance.

So now all the sugar remains in the blood and the insulin is powerless. The pancreas registers the high blood sugar level and because it only knows this schema — too much sugar in the blood, insulin must be produced — it produces even more insulin. Of course, this does not go well for long — at some point it becomes exhausted and gives up. This can eventually result in extremely low, or indeed, no insulin: diabetes. According to the World Health Organization, in 2014 there were 422 million people worldwide suffering from diabetes, the majority of them with type 2 diabetes.

The main risks for type 2 diabetes are poor nutrition, excess weight, and lack of exercise.

A large part of the rejected sugar is kept in the liver as stored sugar, glycogen, or fat. Insulin is also involved in this process; it has an anti-lipolytic action, which means it stops fat cells from being broken down and used as energy. As long as there is insulin in the blood, not a single fat cell will be broken down.

Finally, let's take another look at the trap of 'chronic stress and excess weight', this time from a different angle. The stress hormone cortisol leads to raised blood sugar levels. If the stress does not abate, the same thing happens as in the case of constant food or sugar intake: insulin resistance. The pancreas registers a blood sugar level that is too high and increases production. The pancreas exhausts itself, insulin is lacking and diabetes can develop. It figures, then, that stress reduction (we'll come back to this later) can help to stabilise weight.

GHRELIN — THE HUNGER HORMONE

Ghrelin wasn't discovered until 1999. It sounds reminiscent of the little monster gremlins from the film by the same name. Much like those cute little creatures, ghrelin can be an agent of chaos, causing us to feel hungry more often than is optimal — and causing us to eat more food than our body needs in order to function at its best. But ghrelin can also lessen anxiety and guard against depression.

Ghrelin is formed in many places throughout the body, but it works directly in the brain. It induces the release of growth hormones, and influences our dietary habits, moods, and sleep. Its mode of action is super complex and has not yet been thoroughly researched. It will be interesting to see what surprises research into ghrelin will bring to light in the future.

LEPTIN — THE SATIETY HORMONE

Leptin makes us feel full and is formed by fatty tissue. Leptin is passed into the blood and then reaches the satiety centre of the brain. Leptin also encourages the fat cells to supply the body with energy, thus emptying or shrinking the fat cells.

Failure of the satiety centre to react to leptin is known as leptin resistance. According to the diabetic information service from the Helmholz Institute in 2018, this is the main reason for obesity. Thankfully, it has recently been discovered that exercise can help in cases of leptin resistance.

The thyroid hormones

Inside the body, it can be like a construction site: heavy work is carried out. The building blocks of carbohydrates, fats, and proteins are obtained from our nourishment. These are then used to form and transform cells and tissues, and to initiate processes in the body. Cell waste is removed, components are recycled, energy is gained, and bodily functions are maintained. This is the process of *metabolism*.

Thyroid hormones steer the metabolism the most. They are formed in the thyroid gland, a butterfly-shaped organ in front of the windpipe at the height of the larynx. Like sex hormones, thyroid hormones are subject to a control system that is steered by the brain. The hypothalamus and pituitary gland call the shots here too.

The hypothalamus sends its messenger, thyrotropin-releasing hormone (TRH), to the pituitary gland. This sends thyrotropin-stimulating hormone (TSH) to the thyroid. Once it arrives at the thyroid cells, it facilitates the release of the thyroid hormones T1 to T4. The thyroid hormones are all iodine-containing; their numbering reveals the amount of iodine atoms they have. This is why one of the thyroid's main tasks is the storage of iodine from our food.

Calcitonin, a hormone that lowers the calcium level in our blood, is also formed in the thyroid.

But let's take one thing at a time: the effects of T1 and T2 are still relatively unresearched but could be especially interesting as a therapy option in treating hypothyroidism. We will look at these more closely in Chapter 3.

Only about 10 per cent of T3 is directly produced as an active hormone in the thyroid. If required, it is converted from the inactive storage form, T4 (thyroxin), which makes up 90 per cent of the thyroid hormone. This process of activation (see diagram on page 57) doesn't take place in the thyroid itself, but in the intestine and liver.

If there is enough T3 and T4 circulating in the blood, then the production of TSH from the pituitary gland is stopped. Once more we have a negative reaction that protects the body from overproduction.

T3 and T4 act on every single body cell and operate round the clock. If their level in the blood is in the optimal range, then you will have lots of energy and feel strong, your weight will be stable, and your body will respond relatively swiftly to behavioural changes, such as increased exercise or a healthier diet.

Your hair is shiny and thick, you can regulate your temperature to suit all types of weather and seasons, and your hands are pleasantly warm. Your bowel does what it is required to do without grumbling; there are no problems with your sex life — at least not with your own libido; you have as much energy as you need, and you are enjoying life.

However, if the thyroid hormones are out of sync, then you may experience insomnia, water retention, severe tiredness, digestion issues, lethargy, and depressive moods. Thyroid disorders can also make conception difficult.

In the parathyroid glands, four peanut-sized glands that are situated behind the thyroid in the neck, parathormone (the antagonist of calcitonin) is formed. This promotes bone metabolism and calcium supply.

THYROID HORMONES
Hormones need to be activated!

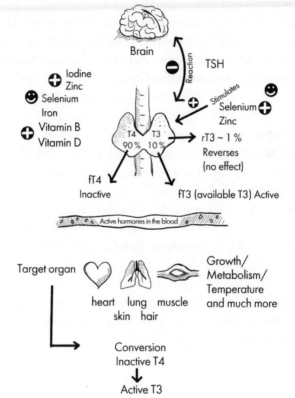

Brain

Reaction

TSH

⊖

➕ Iodine
Zinc
😊 Selenium
Iron
➕ Vitamin B
Vitamin D

Stimulates

➕

Selenium ➕
Zinc

😊

T4   T3
90% 10%

→ rT3 ~ 1 %
Reverses
(no effect)

fT4

Inactive

fT3 (available T3) Active

Active hormones in the blood

Target organ

heart lung muscle
      skin hair

Growth/
Metabolism/
Temperature
and much more

Conversion
Inactive T4
↓
Active T3

T4 —— Conversion ——→ T3
     disrupted by

Stress, gluten, infections,
toxins, diminished bowel
and liver activity

Reverses T3 =
'The rotten twin'
Occupies T3
receptor without
effect

Because the thyroid hormones affect many parts of the body and interact with other hormones, symptoms of hypothyroidism can be complex and varied — so varied that thyroid dysfunction is often not recognised. Statistics from around the world show how serious this is: more than 4 million Germans currently suffer from the form of hypothyroidism known as Hashimoto's thyroiditis, which also affects 1 to 2 per cent of the population in the United States. Women in the phases of hormonal change are particularly susceptible to thyroid disease. As the symptoms can overlap with dysfunction in other glands, we will take a close look at the thyroid in Chapter 3.

Neurotransmitters

Hormones are usually produced in glands and then transported via the blood to other areas, where they take effect. Occasionally they are produced by saliva, or secretions on the spot.

Neurotransmitters are nerve messengers. They allow the nerve cells to communicate with one another by ensuring stimuli are conducted, or blocked, blazingly fast. So, strictly speaking, they are not hormones, even if some of them are known as 'happiness hormones'.

Neurotransmitters are the precursor for some hormones and can have a direct effect on the endocrine glands. But this is not the only reason we discuss them in this chapter and in the book. It's also because they really do make us happy. And we are very much in favour of being happy!

ENDORPHINS — THE NATURAL PAINKILLER

Endorphins are like the body's own morphine; they are messengers with drug-like effects. They are formed in the brain and spinal cord, but also in white blood cells. They have an analgesic effect and dock onto opioid receptors. From this group, beta endorphin (ß) is the substance that has the strongest effect.

In a state of shock, such as after an accident, large amounts of endorphins are produced. They are the reason people with very serious injuries initially don't feel pain, and indeed, often help other victims of an accident. Once that initial flood of endorphins wears off, their body recognises the pain of the injury and then collapses.

Endorphins are also released during stress. Since they act on the same receptors as drugs, it is not surprising that stress can sometimes also lead to euphoria. This is possibly one of the reasons why many people — for example, workaholics — cannot be deterred from their stressful habits. They are addicted to the short-term kick that stress gives them.

DOPAMINE AND SEROTONIN —
THE SOLDIERS OF FORTUNE

The neurotransmitters dopamine and serotonin are produced when we have done something particularly well. This is also known as the reward effect.

Dopamine is the marathon runner. If we are very motivated over a long period of time and have enough drive, then dopamine is responsible. It is formed in the nerve cells in the brain and in the adrenal medulla. Some drugs, such as cocaine, extend the effect of dopamine. Drug consumption satisfies the reward system in the brain, and this is therefore one of the most important triggers for addiction. The dopamine produced in the adrenal medulla is a precursor to the stress hormone noradrenaline.

Lack of dopamine occurs in Parkinson's disease, a disease where movement is typically slowed, and muscular rigidity and tremors occur.

Serotonin is the sprinter that ensures a short-term feeling of happiness. It is formed in the nerve cells of the brain; in thrombocytes, also known as blood platelets; and above all in special cells in the bowel, the enterochromaffin cells. Serotonin is another all-rounder: it affects body temperature and blood pressure, controls our appetite, raises our mood and motivation, acts as a soporific, antidepressant, and relaxant, and encourages the intake of nutrients in the intestine.

The amino acid tryptophan is required for serotonin production. The body cannot produce tryptophan itself, meaning that we have to take it in through our diet.

Chronic stress leads to a malfunction in serotonin metabolism and can result in hypersensitivity, which can lead to aggressive behaviour, anxiety, insomnia, and lack of appetite.

All dopamine and serotonin within the brain must be produced within the brain. There is no alternative. Serotonin from the bowel or dopamine from the adrenal medulla cannot get past the blood–brain barrier. In order for these hormones to be produced by the brain, we really need adequate sleep and good stress-reduction strategies (see Chapter 5 for more on this).

MELATONIN — SLEEP WELL

The sleep hormone melatonin is also produced from serotonin. It is made in the pituitary gland, in the retina, and in the intestine. When the first light of day reaches our eyes, melatonin production is halted, and when it gets dark, production is stimulated. This is how melatonin steers our day–night rhythm.

It makes us feel sleepy by docking onto blood vessels in our brain and immune cells and spreading the message, 'Time to rest now, quieten down, no more eating or playing'.

But it also sends the message, 'Lower the blood pressure and body temperature and fetch the toolbox from the shed'. During the night, the immune system dedicates itself to cell reparation. And the brain secretly continues to learn, and our memory is trained during sleep, so to speak. This is why sleeping long enough and deeply enough is so important.

With increasing age, it is not quite as easy to cultivate this good sleep, as melatonin production begins to decrease from around the age of thirty. This is why issues with insomnia during menopause can be connected to a lack of melatonin.

We were unable to list all the hormones and neurotransmitters in this chapter. As mentioned, there are 150 known ones, and probably thousands of unknown ones. However, the knowledge about the most important hormones and their control circuits that we've outlined allows us to understand most of the symptoms encountered during menopause.

We don't have an answer to all the problems that come with diminishing hormone production, but we do have answers for a large number of them. In the next chapter, the core part of this book, you will read about which products, measures, and tips you can use to support your body and mind. It's going to get really interesting.

3

Balancing Our Hormones — This Is How It Works

Now that we have introduced the hormones, we would like you to fill out our extensive questionnaire. This will help you to gain a better understanding of whether your current physical and/ or psychological experience might indicate a possible hormonal imbalance. Our list of questions is pretty long because hormones affect what is going on in our body and mind in a number of ways. This is why a broad variety of symptoms could all be connected to hormonal disorders.

Time and again it is primarily the most well-known symptoms, like hot flushes, that are linked to hormonal changes. Unfortunately, other symptoms are often misjudged, overlooked, or not taken seriously. Moreover, hot flushes (which can also take the form of night sweats) may have other causes.

It is important to tell your doctor or therapist about your state of health and have the causes checked out.

As you answer the questions, take all the time you need to listen to your body and be honest with yourself about your current state.

This will act as a personal stocktake, which will hopefully help you to reach a better understanding of your own state of health. In this chapter, we will discuss the causes of the individual symptoms in detail and demonstrate which therapies or measures might bring relief.

Our recommendations and tips on hormonal balance and the detailed stocktake of your situation can not only serve as a basis for your discussion with your doctor, but can also help you to activate your 'inner doctor'. We will go into more detail about 'inner doctors' in Chapter 4, where we will show you how you can shape your own personal path in a self-caring and self-determined way. Remember, 'It's not called the "change of life" for nothing.'

We have put the particular hormones that may be out of sync in brackets after the symptoms. The hormone circuits are very complex; we have intentionally limited ourselves to a selection of the main ones. If no state of shortage or dominance (i.e., too much) is noted, then there is an imbalance between certain hormones.

O = Oestrogen (Oestrogen deficiency or oestrogen dominance)
ODE = Oestrogen Deficiency
ODM = Oestrogen Dominance
P = Progesterone
C = Cortisol
T = Testosterone deficiency
HT = Hypothyroidism
I = Insulin
Vit D = Vitamin D

QUESTIONNAIRE

1. Do you suffer from hot flushes — including night sweats? **(ODM, P)**

2. If you are still having periods: do you suffer from PMT? If you do, have these symptoms got worse? **(ODM, P)**

3. If you are still having periods: has your bleeding got worse, more painful, and longer? **(ODM, P)**

4. If you are still having periods: have they become more irregular? **(O, P)**

5. Do you suffer from migraines or cycle-related headaches? **(O, P)**

6. Are you increasingly feeling unrested and excessively tired when you wake up? **(C)**

7. Do feel your energy waning, or a complete loss of energy ('I feel as if my battery has died') or lack of drive? **(ODE, C)**

8. Do your joints ache, particularly in the mornings after you get up, or does your entire body ache ('All my bones are hurting')? **(O, HT)**

9. Do you suffer from muscle tension? **(ODE, HT, Vit D)**

10. Has your muscle strength diminished? **(HT, ODE)**

11. Do you not feel fit enough to do some exercise, or do you feel excessively tired after doing exercise or sport? **(C, ODE)**

12. Have you experienced heart palpitations or cardiac arrhythmia recently? **(O, C, I)**

13. Do you suffer from tachycardia (fast heart rate)? **(O, HT)**

14. Do you have blood circulation issues (a sudden feeling of faintness, weak knees, and dizziness when you stand up)? **(ODE, Vit D, HT, I)**

15. Are you experiencing hair loss or has your hair become dry, brittle, dull, or sparse? **(HT, O)**

16. Has the outer third section of your eyebrows grown sparse or significantly thinner? **(HT)**

17. Are your breasts tender and sore when you touch them? **(ODM, P)**

18. Have your breasts become less full? **(ODE)**

19. Has your cup size gone up recently? **(ODM)**
20. Has your libido decreased significantly ('What was sex again?')? **(T, ODE, ODM, HT)**
21. Is your vagina dry and tender? Does this sometimes cause sex to be painful? **(ODE)**
22. Has your facial hair growth or the amount of hair under your arms increased? **(T)**
23. Do you have sleep issues (getting to sleep or sleeping through the night)? **(C, P, O)**
24. Do you regularly wake up between 1.00 am and 4.00 am? **(O, P)**
25. Is your stomach bloated and do you suffer from constipation? **(HT, ODM, P)**
26. Have you recently started to suffer from allergies or food intolerances? **(ODM, P)**
27. If you are asthmatic, have your symptoms increased? **(ODM)**
28. Has your ability to concentrate diminished? Does your head often feel fuzzy ('brain fog'), as if you were suffering from a hangover but you haven't drunk any alcohol? **(HT, O)**
29. Do you struggle to find the right word or suffer from memory loss? **(O)**
30. Have you become more sensitive to noise? **(O, P, C)**
31. Has your ability to tolerate alcohol diminished? **(O)**
32. Is your face puffy? **(ODM)**
33. If you are still having periods: do you increasingly suffer from water retention (e.g. in your legs), especially shortly before your period? **(O, P)**
34. Have you gained more than five kilograms in the last 12 months, especially around your hips, thighs, and stomach? **(HT, O, P, C, T)**
35. Are you not able to lose weight, or do you lose weight much more slowly than you used to, even though you eat a healthy diet and/or exercise regularly? **(HT, O, P, T)**
36. Have you accumulated fat around your neck? **(C)**
37. Have you been diagnosed with osteoporosis? **(ODE)**

38. Have you been diagnosed with endometriosis or polycystic ovary syndrome? (T, ODM, I)

39. Do you feel emotionally volatile? Are you often irritable? Do you often get flustered or upset? (P, ODM, ODE)

40. Do you feel tearful; are you 'thin skinned'? (O)

41. Do you feel quite down and out of sorts? Are you suffering from a depressive episode or are you taking prescription medication for depression? (ODE, ODM, P, C)

42. Do you suffer from anxiety or panic? Do you worry more and does this keep you awake at night? (P, C, HT, O)

43. Do you struggle to fit all the things you need to do into the day? (T)

44. Do you increasingly feel rushed? (C, O, P)

45. Does the day not have enough hours for all your activities? (C, P, O)

46. Do you feel overwhelmed on several days in the week? (C, HT, O)

47. Do you handle stress less well than you used to? Do stressful situations drain you so that you feel weak and tired afterwards? (HT, C, O, P)

48. Do you generally feel empty and burned out? (C, HT, ODE, P, Vit D)

49. Have you noticed yourself becoming increasingly socially isolated, not going out, not visiting friends or wanting people around you because you need time for yourself? (O, P, HT)

50. Have you been diagnosed with burnout syndrome, or do you suspect you might be experiencing this? (C, HT)

51. Do you often feel that your reaction is inappropriate, that is, that you are reacting unusually or too strongly to a trigger? (O, P, C, HT)

52. Do you feel that you are not as carefree as you used to be? (HT, O, P)

53. Have you lost your zest for life? (HT, O, P)

54. Do you suffer from cold hands and feet? Do you sleep in your socks? **(HT, Vit D, C)**
55. Is your cholesterol too high? **(HT)**
56. Have you been diagnosed with rosacea or redness caused by broken veins in your face? **(ODM)**
57. Have you been having issues with your gallbladder recently? **(ODM)**
58. Have you been diagnosed with fibroids (benign growths in your uterus)? **(O, P)**
59. Have you been diagnosed with cysts in your breasts or ovaries? **(O, P)**
60. Have you been diagnosed with hypothyroidism? **(HT, ODM)**
61. Have you been diagnosed with an autoimmune disorder? **(HT, ODM)**
62. Have you been diagnosed with high blood pressure? **(ODM)**
63. Have fine wrinkles suddenly turned into deep wrinkles ('When did that happen?')? **(ODE)**
64. Do you feel wobbly and weak when you are up and about, especially when you don't eat regularly? **(I)**
65. Do you regularly drink more than two cups of coffee daily or more than four 0.2-litre glasses of alcohol (wine, beer) per week? **(C, O)**
66. Are you addicted to sweet things, carbohydrates, and/or coffee? **(I)**
67. Are you exposed to poisonous substances (toxins) at work? **(O)**
68. Do you regularly eat, daily or several times a week, conventionally sourced meat (i.e. not organic)? **(O)**
69. Do you regularly eat, daily or several times a week, processed foods such as fast food, ready meals, tinned or frozen dishes? **(O)**
70. Do you use cosmetic products or foodstuffs packaged in plastic that contains plasticisers (BPA)? **(O)**

Using our hormones to balance our hormones

Hormones are our managers, personal trainers, counsellors, motivators, beauty team, and much, much more. They inform our cells about the next important steps to take in the body and ensure that they communicate with one another. Maybe this takes place quite unceremoniously: 'Hey, move, hurry up; this way, no, that way; out of the way; move!' Or maybe they speak very respectfully with one another: 'Could you tell Anna that we are out of carbohydrates? Philip, would you like to load the sugar into the cells, please?'

We don't know.

But we do know that without hormones in our body it would be mayhem. We wouldn't be able to go to sleep in the evenings or wake up in the mornings. We wouldn't be able to convert what we eat into energy. We might not even eat, because we simply wouldn't feel hungry. Without the hunger hormone ghrelin as a prompt to stoke up on carbohydrates, fats, and proteins, we would not live for very long.

Hormones are our support team. They give us strength to fight and stamina to flee. They give us happiness, allow us to fall in love, and encourage our feelings of desire for our partner. That is, until they become, well, out of sync.

Our hormones' interplay is often compared to an orchestra. To continue with this analogy: out-of-sync hormones are like someone suddenly playing their own piece instead of the specified score. Too much oestrogen, like at the beginning of perimenopause, would be the flute player who suddenly plays extra notes or tries a new melody. Initially it's only her immediate colleague, the clarinet, who is surprised. She shakes her head at the flute's whims and before you know it, the clarinet has also made a mistake. The violin wonders what's up back there, and ... ouch: her C major has become a C sharp. One after another, the entire orchestra falls out of step.

In this way, a single hormone that is out of sync disrupts all the other hormones. This can have a powerful impact on the body and mind. It would be surprising if it didn't.

When something happens to you in public, it's easy to just shake your head and put it down to hormones going haywire. But you can also — and we think this is the better way — change your own relationship with your little helpers and take up the challenge. Let's see how these 'helpers' can be motivated — maybe a pay rise, a staff outing, a gift basket of nice fruit, or a good book would help?

Ask yourself: how can I support my body? What do I need to be mentally healthy (more on this in Chapter 4)? Even if your female hormones are letting you down right now, in this chapter we will show you how you can bring the team back together. Maybe the team needs reinforcements, or maybe it needs a different type of power food or less stress. A glance around the neighbourhood can also help: off-balance hormones from completely different glands than the ovaries sometimes upset the entire system. These could be hormones from the bowel, for example, or the adrenal glands, and most certainly the thyroid hormones.

SEB: 'As a doctor, I try to look at the symptoms from different angles and get to the bottom what's going on. What is the root of the problem? Looking at the hormone cycle as part of the diagnostic process is essential, in my opinion. Patients often initially seek out their GP when their joints ache or their heart is playing up.

'Doctors enquire much too rarely about a patient's hormonal status — for example, whether she is already in menopause, or is still having periods, whether she is suffering from hot flushes or insomnia, whether she gets out of breath more quickly than she used to, or feels her heart racing, and so on. This comprehensive, holistic approach is hugely important.'

MENOPAUSE: OUR SECOND PUBERTY?

The hormonal change that takes place in our forties is often compared to the one we experience during puberty. There is some truth to this, but if we examine it more closely, the comparison doesn't hold up. During puberty, hormones pipe up; in menopause, they take their leave. It's exactly the opposite situation. This is why the effects of the presence and absence of hormones on the body and mind can't really be seen as similar — apart from the fact that both are extremely challenging phases of life that we have to go through.

> SKB: 'I was 42 when I noticed my body changing. At this time my son was switching from kindergarten to primary school, and I was looking forward to a new period of my life. When he came home with homework, he felt very grown up, and our playtimes with his toys on the carpet, our rides along the bank of the Rhine — him on his balance bike, me on my big bike — our visits to countless playgrounds, were replaced by working side by side at the desk. Of course, we still played, but at different times, and I no longer needed to finish off my articles late at night because I couldn't get to them during the afternoon. Finally, it felt like I had a life in the evenings. But at the same time, I had grown more thin-skinned. I didn't tolerate wine in the evenings as well as I used to, and I suffered from chronic backache for the next five years. I was also very sad to slowly let go of the idea of perhaps ever having a second child.'

Puberty and menopause are both initially characterised by fluctuating hormone levels. When girls start their periods around the age of 12, which is known as the 'menarche', their hormone levels go up and down. It is not until around the age of 20 that the menstrual cycle becomes pretty regular in length and frequency. In your twenties, oestrogen and progesterone levels are at their highest and ensure you have the power and energy to approach life with curiosity, feeling sexy, alert, and energetic. If you stay up all night, the only traces it leaves are dark circles under your eyes, aching muscles from too much dancing, or heartache because it turns out the person you spent the whole night with is already seeing someone. Once you approach your mid-thirties, it's not only your taste in partners and the amount of partying that changes — your body also needs longer to get over things. Disruptions to your system may cause sallow skin, hormonal fluctuations, and cycle disorders. Mental and physical stress, jetlag and/or an unhealthy diet may affect you more than you want to believe. You probably also have a lot on your plate, whether it's your job, your child or children, a new pet, a house move, or relatives that need care or attention. Life becomes busier, fuller, faster. The little detectives in our body realise this: 'Hello! Can anyone hear us?' Probably not. As their host, we are so very busy with life. Before we realise it, ovulation can become more irregular. This is one of the reasons women from their mid-thirties onwards sometimes struggle to get pregnant.

Perimenopause — the beginning

In Germany there are currently about 15 million women between 35 and 55 years old, that is, in their 'prime age' for hormonal changes. Two-thirds of them feel the effects of this — that is about ten million women. It would be cynical of us to claim that if you are one of them, then you are in 'good' company. But you can see there are quite a few of us!

From around the age of 35, so-called 'anovulatory cycles' begin. This means that ovulation does not take place every single month. If you don't pay attention to this, you probably won't even notice; perhaps your periods are a little lighter. Nonetheless, there are consequences: a follicle in which no egg is growing produces less or no progesterone. This causes an imbalance of the two sex hormones. Oestrogen is now, so to speak, out on a limb.

Symptoms in this early period of perimenopause are therefore almost always down to a progesterone deficiency or oestrogen dominance. It is only when you have had no periods for 12 months, are in menopause, and the hormone production in the ovaries has stopped completely, that symptoms of oestrogen deficiency become noticeable. But it may take some time before that happens. Until then, the hormone levels in the blood can fluctuate accordingly. Everything is possible: high oestrogen levels, temporarily low or constantly low levels. Depending on when it begins, this state can continue for 10, 12 or even 15 YEARS.

PROGESTERONE DEFICIENCY —
OR RATHER, OESTROGEN DOMINANCE

Most women (and unfortunately most practitioners too) think that menopausal symptoms are always an oestrogen issue. But in actual fact, the first hormone to take its leave is progesterone. Common symptoms of progesterone deficiency include insomnia, reduced resistance to stress, or a feeling of vague anxiety, as if a grey fog is resting over you. Decreased progesterone levels can also take away our cheerfulness and lightness, and bring about depressive moods. Within the framework of hormone replacement therapy, for many years, progesterone was prescribed solely to protect the uterine lining. This is certainly one therapeutic action of progesterone, but its many other important effects on the mind and nervous systems were shamefully neglected and completely undervalued.

Case study: Progesterone deficiency

Marie, a 41-year-old teacher, was struggling to cope. Everything was getting too much for her, even her much-loved evenings with her girl-friends. She had begun to constantly ask her husband and children to quieten down. Countless little things upset her, and she felt irritable all the time. She didn't recognise or like herself anymore. She'd always been open and extroverted in the past, interested in friends and family and generally very empathetic. Now she just wanted to be alone. Her motto became 'Door locked, phone switched off', so that neither a visitor nor her mobile would disturb her.

Initially, she thought it was just a short phase of exhaustion, which might be connected to the insomnia that she'd recently developed. But then she began to have vague feelings of anxiety and fear. Marie was tired, but the negative thoughts, her permanent state of irritability, and a latent feeling of dissatisfaction wouldn't allow her to find any rest. Marie grew ever sadder, as she loved her family and had, particularly in the last few years, kickstarted several positive career developments. Essentially everything was all right. Except that it wasn't. Marie described it as if she had somehow managed to lose herself.

In Marie's case, it was important to rule out the beginnings of depression, with insomnia and anxiety at the forefront. She had an appointment with a consultant, who ruled this out. Extensive blood tests didn't show any abnormalities; her thyroid function was normal. However, one lab result was conspicuously low: progesterone. Although Marie was still having regular periods, there were already some cycles without ovulation, which were causing progesterone deficiency. The cyclical administration of progesterone capsules at night as well as a change in diet made Marie feel much better. Progesterone has soporific and anxiolytic properties and increases your ability to tolerate stress. Marie started riding again, a sport she had enjoyed a great deal as a child. This helped her to find the 'old' Marie again. Also, knowing that she was in the perimenopausal phase, and being aware of the possible 'traps', had a calming effect on her. She now knew how to take better care of herself in the future.

In this first part of perimenopause — although this can, as we already said, last for what seems like an eternity — the following symptoms may occur or become worse:

- PMS
- Bleeding between periods
- Heavier and longer periods
- Increased growth of the uterine lining
- Growth of benign tumours, fibroids in the uterus
- Stronger mood fluctuations
- Headaches, migraines
- Tiredness
- Bloating
- Shortness of breath, especially during exercise
- Weight increase
- Water retention
- Irritability (aggression, quick temper)
- Low stress tolerance

- Insomnia
- Depressive moods
- Various types of cancer (breast cancer, ovarian cancer)
- Increased risk of autoimmune disease (Hashimoto's disease)

If you have asthma, high oestrogen levels like those in the days before your period can also cause severe attacks. This is described as 'perimenstrual asthma'. Oestrogen-related asthma symptoms increase in a third of pregnant patients as well as women in perimenopause. If you have asthma, do inform your doctor or consultant if you are taking the pill or other hormones. Your hormones may need to be adapted to the medication (allergy or asthma medication), or vice versa. It may make sense for asthma patients who take hormones to have their hormone levels checked.

Another serious topic is headaches and migraines that can be caused or intensified by an oestrogen dominance. Women who experience migraines tend to suffer from more frequent attacks when their hormones are out of balance. Give progesterone a try; in many cases this rebalances the hormones and reduces symptoms. In addition, we also recommend that those suffering from headaches take 300 milligrams of magnesium, both morning and night. This counteracts cramping in the vascular muscles. If your faeces become softer, then reduce the dose to 300 milligrams per day.

If you have an office job or spend a lot of time at your computer, pay attention to your eyes. Lengthy, fixed staring at a screen is like high-performance sport for your eyes, and is extremely tiring. This can also encourage headaches. You may find it helps if you do eye exercises in between sessions at the computer, or if you get a pair of reading glasses designed for screen work — especially if you already use reading glasses.

These are our tips when headaches or migraines increase during hormone replacement therapy.

STRESS STEALS HORMONES

The pregnenolone burglary

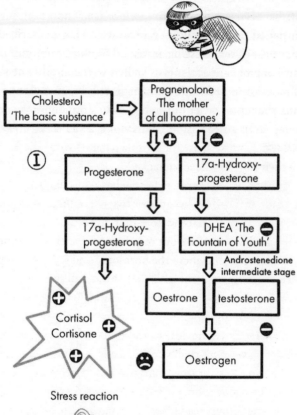

Cholesterol 'The basic substance' → Pregnenolone 'The mother of all hormones'

① Progesterone (+)

17a-Hydroxy-progesterone (−)

17a-Hydroxy-progesterone

DHEA 'The Fountain of Youth' (−)

Androstenedione intermediate stage

Oestrone | testosterone

Cortisol Cortisone (+) (+) (+)

Oestrogen (−)

Stress reaction

Hormone shift towards stress
Pregnenolone is 'kidnapped' towards ①

Progesterone deficiency, or oestrogen dominance, can also be caused by factors other than decreasing ovulation. Hypothyroidism during perimenopause, which occurs in approximately 30 per cent of women, may be connected to progesterone deficiency. Similarly, endocrine disruptors such as plasticisers (see Chapter 4), as well as stress, also encourage this imbalance. Important precursors, essential to the formation of progesterone, are simply stolen to produce the stress hormone cortisol. The most important precursor is pregnenolone, which is also known as the 'mother of all steroid hormones' (see illustration on page 77). Pregnenolone increases memory function, helps our resilience to stress, improves our mood, and encourages sleep. Stress carries out a so-called 'pregnenolone burglary'.

Fibroids

At some point in their lives, half of all women develop benign growths in their uterus: fibroids. These benign tumours very rarely develop into cancer. They can remain relatively small for years and not cause any problems. But with the start of perimenopause, they can significantly increase in size due to an oestrogen surplus. This is why they are usually found in women over 40. After menopause, they often shrink again, as if (almost) nothing happened. Depending on where they are located within the wall of the uterus, they can cause prolonged, heavy, and often painful periods. They can also cause bleeding between periods, pain, and/or unpleasant pressure in the lower abdomen and pelvis. You may need to go to the toilet more often, as depending on the length and size of the fibroids, they may put pressure on your bladder. The size of your stomach may grow without you having gained any weight. Fibroids can also cause backache.

If your periods are heavy or if you regularly experience bleeding between periods, then you may develop an iron deficiency caused by the blood loss. This may cause feelings of physical weakness and your mental capacity may also decrease, which can cause concentration difficulties.

It is important to note here that increased bleeding, bleeding between periods, and bleeding that occurs after menopause need to be checked with a gynaecologist in order to rule out other causes.

Case study: Fibroids

Sabrina, an ear, nose, and throat consultant, was 41. She had suffered from painful and long, heavy periods for many years. She was completely exhausted by the time she sought help. Large fibroids were discovered during a clinical examination. The gynaecologist who was treating Sabrina advised her to have a hysterectomy. After the operation, Sabrina was prescribed hormone treatment. A few weeks after the operation, she came to my surgery and complained of strong mood swings, a deep sadness she'd never felt before, and a vague feeling of anxiety. Sabrina, who was normally so confident and who had previously easily managed all her work challenges, seemed intimidated and tearful.

We had a lengthy conversation about the impact of the operation. Her job had always come first. She had built up a large practice, spent a lot of time with her friends and her samba group, and had been very happy without a family of her own. She had never really wanted children, but the hysterectomy had brought it home to her that this was now firmly off the agenda. We spent a long time talking about the physical intervention, but also about the mental impact, and the sadness and fear that came with it. I also asked Sabrina about the name of her hormone medication. To my surprise (and horror), I discovered that she had been prescribed an oestrogen product and no progesterone. This really was very oldschool. Following a hysterectomy, progesterone is anything but redundant, even if its powers of protecting the uterine lining are no longer needed. Nowadays, women are given a form of bioidentical progesterone following a hysterectomy. This works as an antidepressant and has an anxiolytic and soporific effect. I am quite sure that alongside the emotional and physical burden that came with the operation, as well as an iron deficiency, a hormone imbalance — in this case a lack of progesterone — was a key contributor to Sabrina's symptoms.

We already mentioned in Chapter 1 that for many years, a hysterectomy was the standard operation for women going through menopause. It is the most frequently performed major gynaecological operation in the world. In 2012, one woman in six in Germany between the age of 18 and 79 had had their uterus removed; a 2017 study found that in Australia, one in three women over the age of 45 had undergone the procedure. The ovaries were also often removed during the operation, which was mostly justified as a preventative measure to avoid possible tumours.

The medical term for the operation is *hysterectomy*. Let's savour that name slowly. It originates from the Greek word *hystera*, meaning 'uterus', and was specifically selected because it was considered proven that women were no longer 'hysterical' after the removal of their uterus! At the beginning of the 20th century, hysteria was considered a typical female affliction. When women showed signs of mental distress and disturbed behaviour, they were diagnosed as a psychiatric illness. Thousands of women were committed to institutions for this reason. 'Madness was female' was the title of an article on this subject in the *Süddeutsche Zeitung* a few years ago. Of course, it wasn't. In the first place, the diagnosis resulted from the fragmented knowledge that doctors had of the female body: when women stopped 'functioning' at around a certain age, then the uterus was blamed. 'You can't have children anymore anyway, so be happy that you got rid of this superfluous organ,' was the send-off that a doctor gave a patient in a clinic here in Germany last year.

The uterus is anything but superfluous. Removing it, and especially removing the ovaries, has far-reaching consequences for hormone production. And even if the ovaries are not removed, tying off vessels and nerves in the pelvis results in slowly killing off the things they supply. The patient goes into menopause. The risk of osteoporosis, strokes, and cardiovascular disease increases. The tissue hormone produced by the uterus, which services the heart and blood vessels, is suddenly gone, as are its positive effects on these parts of the body. Because the hormone-like substances that are important for the contraction of the uterine muscles are no longer present, emotional regulation can also be affected. This is why hysterectomies have been linked to anxiety and depression. Loss of sensation in the pelvis, incontinence, reduced libido, and less intense orgasms are additional ramifications. Anyone surprised?

This of course leads to the question, what can you do about fibroids apart from surgery?

Medication

Two approved medications are available for the treatment of fibroids: analogues of GnRH (gonadotropin-releasing hormone) and the selective UPA (ulipristal acetate, a progesterone receptor modulator). Both stop menstruation within days or weeks and, if they are taken over a long period of time, the fibroid tissue shrinks. Given their side effects on the liver, though, these medications should not be taken for too long. Liver function values need to be checked regularly while on either of them.

Focused ultrasound

Specialised ultrasound therapy is a relatively new fibroid treatment. It can only be used to treat small fibroids of an eight-centimetre diameter or less. The tissue is treated using a focused high-energy ultrasound, which ablates the tumour. The chance of success is said to be around 80 per cent. This method is only available in certain clinics.

Dietary changes and weight loss

Even a weight loss of just 5 per cent — say, from 65 to 62 kilograms — could have a positive effect on the growth of fibroids. This is because fat tissue produces oestrogen — so, less fat tissue means less oestrogen. In order to limit the danger of inflammation, it is worth making dietary changes and avoiding consuming milk products and meat. The pro-inflammatory arachidonic acid contained in meat can intensify painful periods. Animal products also contain hormones (see the section on nutrition) that may encourage fibroid growth.

Compounds

Magnesium relaxes the muscles and can alleviate pain. In cases of acute symptoms, you can take 100 milligrams orally every hour, up to a maximum dose of 600 milligrams. If your faeces become softer, then lower the dose.

Iron: in the case of anaemia caused by increased or more frequent bleeding, iron levels should be monitored regularly, and a possible deficiency addressed by taking a supplement.

A hysterectomy can bring relief, and can be necessary for women who have severe pain, bleeding, or problems during urination. However, we would like every woman to be fully informed about the benefits, implications, and risks of such a big operation. So, we ask you not to allow yourself to be bounced into it. If your mother or grandmother had a hysterectomy, this does not automatically mean that you also need one. Only one in ten hysterectomies is due to a cancer diagnosis. Provided you do not have cancer, we would encourage you to consider very carefully, together with your gynae-cologist, the implications of removing this important organ.

Perimenopause — in the thick of it

We have spent a long time discussing progesterone deficiency, or rather oestrogen surplus, and maybe you are wondering: when are they going to get around to talking about hot flushes?

These occur when oestrogen diminishes. This is usually the case when you are in your mid-to-late forties or early fifties, but sometimes earlier. Oestrogen deficiency can cause acute symptoms, but it can also have long-term serious effects later on, such as an increased risk of osteoporosis, cardiovascular disease, and some forms of cancer.

But back to the hot flushes. They are often the first symptom of menopause and can continue for up to five years (and in rarer cases, up to ten years) after menopause.

HOT FLUSHES

This menopausal classic besets 90 per cent of us. Hot flushes vary from person to person. They usually do not cause any body odour, take a few seconds or several minutes, and can occur sporadically or up to 20 times a day. They may spread across your chest and neck, or across your face. In addition to the feeling of warmth or sweating, the skin may redden significantly and be accompanied by heart palpitations and dizziness. This can be scary, especially the first time it happens. Often you don't know what is going at first.

> SEB: 'Many of my patients don't realise that they are having hot flushes, especially if these happen earlier than expected and don't correspond to the stereotype. For example, a slim, sporty, young patient asked me how much it would cost to inject Botox into her sweat glands. She had read about this treatment method for excessive sweating. When questioned, it turned out that she wasn't sweating in those areas where Botox is usually injected, namely under your armpits. Hot

flushes usually spread across the chest and face. This patient didn't need Botox — she was 39 years old, was in a stressful phase of her life, and already in perimenopause.

'In my case it wasn't very different. I had a phase during which I often woke up at night feeling very hot. I assumed this was a sign of viral infection or a worse chronic infection. It became clear to me that it was something else when on a long drive one day in early summer I thought I'd mistakenly put on the seat heating. The hot flush manifested itself as a strong feeling of warmth in the middle of my back. It was ten in the morning, and the rental car didn't even have heated seats! A few weeks later — as often happens in perimeno-pause — my body resumed its hormone production. The sweating disappeared just as quickly as it had come. Until the next hormonal decline.'

Hot flushes are caused by a steepening hormonal decline, which among other things causes a system error in the central thermo-regulation in the brain. It's as though the thermostat on the heater is playing up, cranking up the heat full blast in the living room at seemingly random times, regardless of whether it's day or night.

As warmth is followed by cold, some women wake up at night. They are drenched in sweat and feel cold or even start shivering because their sweat-dampened skin has cooled off. Some women have to change their nightwear several times during a night. Others don't sweat at all during the night, only during the day. But this can be so excessive that they get damp patches on their clothes. This cliché keeps reappearing in films and television programs — the menopausal woman is made a mockery of. But, of course, it's not funny — especially if you have a job in which you deal with people, such as teacher to a class of pubescent 16-year-olds, for example. And definitely not if the hot flushes are accompanied by other non-specific symptoms, such as a feeling of pressure in your head or chest, restlessness, nausea, heart palpitations, or shortness of breath.

You may have been having hot flushes for many years, which have been very tedious and which you could well have done without. Some people find that their symptoms improve when they limit their consumption of coffee, black tea, alcohol, and spicy, rich, hot foods. As well as adjusting your diet in this way, you can also try doing anything you can to reduce your stress levels, sleeping in a cooler room, and wearing breathable fabrics.

One age-old home recipe against sweating is sage tea. The essential oils in sage inhibit sweat production. Drink several cups a day. Alternating hot and cold footbaths and showers may bring relief. Acupuncture also helps a lot of women.

Classic antidepressants help 60 per cent of women. But we do not want to recommend this as the only treatment for hot flushes. In 95 per cent of women who have hormone replacement therapy (either conventional hormone replacement or bioidentical hormone therapies), the hot flushes disappear (see pages 101 and 103).

Apart from hot flushes, so many other symptoms can be triggered by an oestrogen deficiency that sometimes it is hard to see the wood for the trees:

- Irritability (tearful, thin-skinned)
- Restlessness
- Mood swings
- Insomnia
- Forgetfulness
- Struggling to find words
- Dry skin and mucous membranes
- Dry eyes (if you can no longer tolerate your contact lenses, this may be linked to an oestrogen deficiency)
- Thinning skin
- Hair loss
- Increased wrinkles
- Urinary tract infections
- Urge to urinate

- Arrhythmia (irregular heartbeat)
- Decreased blood circulation in the vagina
- Vaginal infections
- Stress incontinence (increased urination)
- Increase in facial hair
- Slackening or shrinking breast tissue
- Inability to conceive
- Depressive moods
- Increased appetite
- Weight gain
- Osteoporosis
- Arteriosclerosis
- Cardiovascular disease
- Change in vaginal flora

Case study: A partner's experience

SEB: 'I interviewed my friend Beate's husband for this book because I think it is important to get a partner's perspective too. How might hormone fluctuations affect relationships? How do men deal with it? Peter really impressed me in this respect. He said that, at first, he'd felt like he'd lost his wife to menopause. I thought that was a strong, honest and touching comment.

'Peter didn't really pick up on it when his wife first started to experience hormonal changes. When Beate started getting annoyed about things that previously wouldn't have upset her, he initially thought it was because she was over-worked or experiencing stress in the office. Then she started getting tearful, and he couldn't talk her into going out in the evenings. She was tired or irritated — sex was out of the question — and there was no chance of intimacy. Eventually Peter became convinced that Beate was suffering from depression. His brother-in-law had been treated in a clinic for several weeks for severe depression a few years previously, which is where Peter got this idea from.

'He spoke to Beate about his worries, and they came to see me in my surgery. With the help of a specialist colleague, I was able to rule out depression; it was clear to me that her symptoms were actually linked to hormonal changes. I encouraged Beate to confide in her gynaecologist at her next appointment. He prescribed bioidentical hormones for her, which stabilised her condition. I admired Peter for the way he had sought out a solution together with his wife during this difficult period in their relationship.

'In my opinion, a lot of instances in which women are treated with antidepressants are not attributable to a mental health issue or sudden exhaustion, but to a change in hormonal balance. So, in my opinion you always need to look at the hormonal cycle when coming to a diagnosis.'

Hormonal imbalance during perimenopause is often caused by a testosterone deficiency. The focus here is primarily on DHEA, the 'Fountain of Youth' hormone, which we explored back in Chapter 2. A DHEA deficiency can manifest as tiredness, insomnia, loss of strength, thinning skin, loss of libido, diminishing body and pubic hair, osteoporosis, hot flushes, and anaemia due to a decrease in the formation of red blood cells. It can also lead to depressive moods, anxiety, nervousness, and irritability. If DHEA levels are measured and there is found to be a deficiency, this can be treated with hormone replacement therapy.

Menopause

The word *menopause* actually describes an end and not a pause; it really does have to be phrased that drastically — even if in Latin the word *pausa* means both an interruption and an end. 'Menopause' is used to describe a hormonal change that lasts for years and that is labelled as such only after the event. The diagnosis happens only in hindsight — when you have not had a period for 12 months, the final period was menopause. At this point, there is only minimal hormone production; fatty tissue and adrenal glands take on a small part of the ovaries' tasks. It is only after menopause that you no longer require contraception, and it is only now that oestrogen and progesterone decline permanently.

This is why most people (including doctors) don't look at the symptoms earlier. And this could be after many women have spent up to 15 years dealing with the whole perimenopausal hassle. So here comes our plea again: remember that physical and mental symptoms in your early forties could be connected to hormonal changes!

Oestrogen deficiency can also occur in women with anorexia, extremely athletic people, those who have disorders in the superior hormone centres of the pituitary gland and hypothalamus, or very rarely, in people with a genetic predisposition. The hormone circuit control also cuts off oestrogen production during breastfeeding. Nature came up with this mechanism in order to protect the body from getting pregnant again too quickly. However, nature is capricious and so breastfeeding is not recommended as a form of contraception.

> SEB: 'The much-vaunted contraceptive method of breastfeeding presented me with beautiful twin girls 18 months after the birth of my son.'

In many women, the only hormone that does not decline, even in old age, is testosterone. As it is no longer balanced out by the other sex hormones, it is described as a testosterone or androgen surplus. This also occurs in young women with PCOS (polycystic ovary syndrome — an enlargement of the ovaries with increased production of male hormones); this condition can affect fertility and make it difficult to conceive. Acne, marked weight gain (obesity), and an increased risk of type 2 diabetes, arteriosclerosis, and high blood pressure, as well as lipid metabolic disorder, can also be linked to this surplus. In addition, there may be increased hair growth around your chin, face, and body. You can also start losing hair on your head. Emotionally, you may feel agitated and aggressive. This can all be extremely challenging for many women.

Before we go into more detail about hormone therapy, we would like to suggest that you speak to your mother or other relatives about their experience with menopause. A mother's age when she began menopause will have some bearing on her child's experience too. Some of my patients and friends have described turbulent times in the family home when they were growing up. It is also worth taking another look at events from a hormonal perspective when examining crises between mothers and adult daughters. Which physical or mental changes did you perceive in your mother? What support did your mother get? Was there an open exchange with friends, doctors, or other relatives? What approaches to this time of life might you have consciously or unconsciously inherited from your mother? If your father was present during this time, how did he deal with the situation?

Reflecting on these questions could significantly influence the way you approach your own menopause. We will come back to this in Chapter 4.

Hormone therapy

In medicine, hormones are used on a daily basis to save lives. For example, cortisone, the inactive form of cortisol, is used for acute allergic shock or asthma attack, and the supply of insulin is essential for many diabetics.

Nonetheless, the subject divides people. The first thing many people hear about hormones is usually in connection with food scandals (hormones in meat), doping, or bodybuilding — in other words, in the context of terrible side effects through misuse or wrongdoing. But as is so often the case, it is worth staying open, and not making a summary rejection based on just a few popular facts and stories. And of course, for those women entering menopause who have been on the contraceptive pill at some point in their lives, taking hormones is nothing new.

Hormone replacement therapy is an option for women in menopause who are experiencing symptoms. In order to understand what we are talking about in this chapter — including the discussion about the pros and cons of hormone replacement therapy, especially in connection with an increased cancer risk — it is important to know that there are two different types of treatment: synthetic and bioidentical. The current trend is towards bioidentical hormones. Let's take a closer look at the differences.

Synthetic and conjugated hormones

In the 1960s, scientists began to obtain oestrogen from the urine of pregnant mares for the purposes of hormone replacement therapy (HRT), or to produce synthetic hormones. These hormones are also known as conjugated oestrogens, which means they are a mixture of hormones.

These hormone-like substances are not structurally identical to endogenous hormones (those you make within your own body). They usually have a stronger and longer effect. The normal dose of synthetic oestrogen can make the concentration of oestrogen six times higher than the natural oestrogen level of a premenopausal woman.

Synthetic oestrogens have a different chemical structure from endogenous hormones, and they are also broken down and converted to other substances. These in turn affect our system in ways that are quite different from the metabolic products of endogenous oestrogen. The immediate metabolic products of the synthetic hormone often cause interference, because the body does not have the right tools — or rather, the right enzyme system — to further use them or dispose of them. Also, the feedback mechanism to the endogenous hormone production is suppressed; there is no longer any communication between the pituitary gland (in the brain) and the ovaries, because there is enough oestrogen in the body.

As a rule, synthetic hormones are stronger and, as they are taken in the form of a pill, they need to be metabolised via the intestine and the liver. The liver is strongly challenged, and the gall bladder also has to rev up its engine quite a bit. Because oestrogens consist of cholesterol, that is, fat, more bile acid is required to reduce the fat. This oestrogen breakdown can lead to increased clotting factors in the liver. This increases the danger of blood clots, thrombosis, and embolisms. There is also an increased risk of gall stones and excessive cholesterol.

Synthetic progesterone-like substances are generally described as *gestagens*. So, when we go on to talk about gestagens, we always mean the artificial replacement for endogenous progesterone. Gestagens were first developed in a laboratory, when it became clear that using synthetic oestrogens on their own resulted in a significantly increased risk of cervical cancer. The active substances are *drospirenone*, *levonorgesterel*, and *medroxyprogesterone acetate (MPA)*, which as antagonists to oestrogen, prevent an excessive build-up of the uterine lining. However, gestagens often only cover a small, very limited part of the function of endogenous progesterone.

Before we discuss hormone products for menopause, we would

first like to talk about a synthetic hormone product that everyone is familiar with: the pill.

Most women are not aware that the pill is a synthetic hormone that significantly intervenes in the hormone cycle. It uses the negative feedback mechanism of follicle-stimulating hormone-oestrogen. You could say it tricks this mechanism through its high content of oestrogen and gestagens (or only gestagens): 'Hey, pituitary gland: there are enough hormones in the blood. This means we are pregnant. Cut down on FSH production.'

So, the pituitary gland can take time off, or at least it no longer has to produce FSH and LH (that's luteinising hormone, which stimulates ovulation) in order to allow an egg cell to develop. This is why ovulation then does not take place — the contraceptive effect works perfectly.

We know from many studies over the last few years that receptors for endogenous progesterone can be found not only in the uterus but also in many organs and tissues in the body, including the brain. These are different from synthetic gestagens. This is why endogenous progesterone influences the metabolism and the action of the thyroid hormones. In contrast to gestagens, endogenous progesterone also has a positive effect on our mood. The endogenous hormone acts as an anxiolytic and an antidepressant. It also helps us to sleep and improves our ability to tolerate stress. In the fertile years, the greatest amount of progesterone is formed in the corpus luteum following ovulation. But when the pill prevents ovulation, the effect of the endogenous progesterone is missing.

It is enormously important for young women to live out their own sexuality without worrying about getting pregnant, and there's no arguing that the pill allows this. However, the pill can also disrupt the body's natural feeling. Many women experience a drop in their libido when taking the pill, and only discover their natural desire after they stop taking it.

One of the reasons that some women's desires can be curbed when taking the pill is the fact that the synthetic hormone can change their sense of smell: this can mean that women are unable to smell their sexual partner in the same way as before. Their own body scent can also change.

In saying all this, we are in no way questioning the purpose of the pill. However, there are studies that show that a high percentage of women take the pill for reasons other than contraception. Also, many people start taking the pill from the age of 13 or 14. This is why, alongside the revolutionary freedom that the pill provides, it is important to know that it radically interferes in the body's natural hormonal balance and can cause side effects such as thrombosis, pulmonary embolism, weight gain, water retention, headaches, vaginal infections, spotting, mood swings, mild to severe depression, anxiety, and panic attacks. If someone is experiencing any of these symptoms, it's a sign that the pill they're taking is not right for them.

In most cases, women take the pill continuously for ten, 15, or 20 years, until they want to get pregnant. During this lengthy period of time, their individual cycle is suspended, so it can take a while for the body to find its way back to its original rhythm. In some cases, the interplay between the ovaries and the brain is so drastically affected that the natural balance is never restored. Failure to conceive then leads people to a fertility clinic, in which the long-immobilised ovaries have to be awoken from their deep slumber.

> SEB: 'When we were prescribed the pill as young women, many of us didn't ask about what was in it and assumed that everything would be fine. Today I ask myself why it took me so long to understand what the pill actually is and what effects it has on the body: these are synthetic substances that intervene massively and block the hormone cycles, sometimes permanently! What is probably the most important side effect is reasonably well known — the increased danger

of thrombosis, especially in smokers. I vaguely remember
my doctor explaining to me that the pill creates a sort of
artificial pregnancy in the body and that this process brought
about the contraceptive effect. At the time, that was enough
for me.

'It's incomprehensible and also irresponsible that young
women are being prescribed the pill purely to suppress symptoms such as acne or painful periods. In particular, young
girls from the age of 14 upwards are given the pill without
proper consideration of the risks. I often have students in
my waiting room suffering from migraines, who are feeling
depressed and lethargic, or who have gained a significant
amount of weight and are suffering the consequences.'

According to data from one of Germany's leading insurance
companies, 11 per cent of female children aged 12–15 and 60 per
cent of those aged 16–20 take the pill. These young girls are often
prescribed the pill because they have irregular cycles and skin problems. In some of these cases, the cause could be polycystic ovary
syndrome (PCOS). PCOS is a metabolic disorder usually combined
with insulin resistance and excess weight, as well as altered thyroid
hormones, and androgen imbalance. Because PCOS can be treated
by medications other than the pill as well as by an appropriate diet,
this is worth considering.

Isolated acne can also be treated in other ways, such as external
intensive cosmetic treatments or a short-term course of antibiotics.
The complexion often improves significantly if the patient avoids dairy
and meat products. Restoring the intestinal flora can also be effective.

At the moment, there is a wave of pill-weariness. On the one hand,
women don't want to have to think about contraception every day,
but nor do they want to think about synthetic hormones circulating around their body. Many women who take the pill suffer side
effects and don't feel comfortable in their bodies: they feel bloated,

different, strange. As a contraceptive method for young women, we would like to mention another hormone-free solution, other than condoms: the small copper-coil IUD that is embedded in the uterine wall like a piercing, or a copper-pearl ball that is positioned in the uterus by a gynaecologist. Both release copper ions that have a two-fold contraceptive effect: they paralyse the sperm, and also slightly irritate the uterine lining, so that a fertilised egg cannot embed itself. The copper coil is recommended for older women, and after giving birth, many women have an IUD fitted. But you could certainly discuss this option and others with your gynaecologist no matter what your age.

As a mature woman, you have to deal with the issue of contraception right up until menopause. If you do not wish to get pregnant, there is no avoiding it. Right up to your very last period there is a minute chance that an egg may be fertilised. The hormonal therapies that we are about to introduce as treatment for menopausal symptoms are *not* a replacement for the pill — in other words, they do not protect you from unwanted pregnancy! Discuss the issue of contraception with your gynaecologist if you no longer want to take the pill.

HORMONE REPLACEMENT THERAPY — HRT

All drugs have side effects. This applies to the pill as well as all other hormone treatments. Because the increased risk of cancer through HRT is the main concern for those considering taking hormones to deal with menopausal symptoms, this is the concern we would like to address first.

Let's start this controversial topic with a quote: 'HRT is the most effective treatment method for the symptoms of menopausal, perimenopausal, and postmenopausal women ... cancer risks are not usually a reason to advise against the therapy.' This is what Olaf Ortmann, the president of the German Cancer Society and head of the Clinic for Gynaecology and Obstetrics at the University Regensburg Hospital, said at the congress of the German Society for Gynaecology and Obstetrics (DGGG) in 2018.

In practice, there is still a great deal of concern among doctors and women who are considering HRT. The reason for this concern is highlighted in a single study, the Women's Health Initiative (WHI) study, which we will come to in a moment.

Breast tissue reacts sensitively to oestrogens and other hormones. You might notice this if your breasts swell just before your period each month because of the raised level of oestrogen.

Hormones make breast tissue grow — that's plausible. And at the same time, we know that breast cancer is the most prevalent malignant tumour in women. But let's take a look at how the DGGG assesses the cancer risk in its most recent guidelines:

- Breast cancer: Out of 10,000 women taking combined HRT (oestrogen and gestagens) over a period of five years, an extra two per year will develop breast cancer. Once HRT has been discontinued, within two to three years the risk of breast cancer drops to the same level as that of a woman who hasn't taken any hormones. (Note: this describes a remote risk. Nobody should develop cancer, and the word 'remote' is of course always meaningless if you are the one affected. Nonetheless, this is the assessment of the risk. The same also goes for ovarian cancer.)
- Ovarian cancer: out of 10,000 women taking combined HRT, an extra nine will be affected per year.
- Endometrial cancer: the risk under HRT is raised only if not enough gestagens or progesterone are taken to protect the uterine lining. If these are taken for ten to 12 days per month, then the risk is *not* elevated.
- Bowel cancer: the risk under HRT is verifiably *lowered* by half when women take hormones for nine to 14 years.

- Women who develop or have had a hormone-dependent cancer should *not* be given HRT, as this increases the risk of a relapse. However, in those cancer patients whose quality of life is severely affected by symptoms of menopause, the DGGG recommends HRT in exceptional cases.

The protection of the uterine lining through progesterone treatment is undeniably important. As breast cancer often appears during the phase of a woman's life when progesterone levels have reduced significantly, further research is needed to show whether taking progesterone might not only protect the uterine lining, but also protect the breast tissue. Progesterone tells the cells: 'Stop growing now, that's enough, and there are enough of you.' In medical terms, this means that it encourages cell development and reduces cell division. Both protect against prolific growth, a peculiarity of cancer cells.

Hormones are a factor in several types of cancer, but we now know that cancer can be triggered by many other factors, for example through lack of exercise, excess weight, genetic predisposition, smoking, alcohol, animal proteins etc.

Therefore, we would very much like to see an end to the scaremongering around hormone replacement therapy and for discussions around the topic to be more objective — especially as new low-dosage hormone treatments and bioidentical formulae are now available.

When women suffer from severe menopausal symptoms, no longer feel like themselves, and have low energy levels — and when this state can exacerbate serious physical ailments such as osteoporosis — then fuelling the fear of breast cancer is not only unhelpful, but also counterproductive. That's why we would emphatically like to make the case for a continuously controlled and personalised hormone therapy with bioidentical products — with proper assessment of the risks and benefits.

A study and its repercussions

The history of hormone replacement therapy is characterised by trials and tribulations. In particular, HRT fell into disrepute because of the initial results of a study carried out by the WHI in 2002. In the years that followed, the prescription rate for HRT products went down by 70 per cent. We would like to point out that in 2016, 14 years later, the original researchers who carried out this study apologised for a misinterpretation of their data and the uncertainty that accompanied it. For 'uncertainty' read: 'inciting panic and fear among thousands of women and doctors!'

They did actually apologise — and we can assure you that this has rarely happened in the history of science. Professor of gynaecology Matthias Wenderlein, from the University Clinic Ulm, put it quite bluntly in the *Deutsche Ärzteblatt* in 2017: 'The negative reports from the WHI on hormone replacement are history.'

What sort of study was it? The initial idea wasn't bad. They wanted to find out: is HRT beneficial? Does it protect women from cardiovascular symptoms? Do they feel better?

As always when you want to prove something in medicine, you work with comparison groups, the bigger the better. You need one group that is given the compound, and one that isn't, or rather one group that *thinks* they have been given medication. The power of the mind to respond to a placebo should not be underestimated.

No sooner said than done: 16,000 women aged between 50 to 79 (average age: 63) were included in the WHI study for an indefinite period of time. The main focus was on the risk of breast cancer and cardiovascular disease. Half the women were given an oestrogen compound derived from the urine of pregnant mares, combined with gestagens; the other group was given a placebo.

The experiment went on for a good ten years, until it was terminated in 2002 for ethical reasons. More of the women in the HRT group developed breast cancer and had heart attacks, strokes, and pulmonary embolisms than those in the placebo group. A disaster!

However, today we can see that the approach to the study was wrong from the start. This was not done intentionally, but out of ignorance. Many of the participants had had menopause for too long before they started taking HRT — in some cases their last period had been 20 years earlier. This meant that the window of opportunity, the favourable time frame for hormone replacement, had been missed in most of the study participants. Later studies were able to show that starting HRT early had a positive effect on the arteries and therefore protected people from cardiovascular diseases.

The second weak spot was in the synthetic hormones themselves, as they bore little resemblance to the hormones they were supposed to be replicating. And the third: the synthetic hormones were given in a very high dosage. Over the years, dosages of synthetic hormones have been continuously reducing. A modern hormone replacement today ideally supplies the body with exactly the amount that it needs in order to carry out its functions. Modern HRT is individually adapted for the patient's personal medical history, their current symptoms, and how long they have experienced these.

Window of opportunity

We now know that hormone therapy, meaning the administration of *replacement* hormones, should begin early — that is, when the first symptoms such as hot flushes appear. This can be around the age of 50, but it could also occur in a person's late thirties. In any case, HRT needs to be started within ten years of the last period, as it is only then that it not only mitigates hot flushes and other acute, early symptoms, but also offers proven protection from long-term, serious illnesses such as osteoporosis, dementia, bowel cancer, and cardiovascular disease (including heart attacks and strokes).

This is the crux of our message: do not suffer for five or ten years before you decide on hormone replacement therapy. Don't let yourself be fobbed off. If necessary, keep badgering your doctor. Discuss the risks that rule out hormone replacement therapy in your case.

For example, if you have had thrombosis or a pulmonary embolism in the past, or suffer from gall bladder or liver disease, or oestrogen-sensitive forms of cancer such as ovarian, breast, or cervical cancer, then you shouldn't take *any* hormones. This also applies if your menopause was more than ten years ago. In exceptional cases, the therapy needs to be carefully gauged and strictly monitored.

If you decide to take hormones, then two forms of hormone replacement therapy are available to you:

Conventional Hormone Replacement Therapy (HRT)

For decades now, a synthetic oestrogen compound that contains conjugated oestrogens has been used to treat menopausal symptoms after menopause has begun.

As mentioned, the chemical structure is not identical to human oestrogen, and this is why its by-products also have non-bioidentical chemical structures. These often create highly unfavourable extraneous substances that swim through our bloodstream. The concentration and the duration of effectiveness are also completely different.

When these treatments are taken orally, the brain–ovary hormone control circuit is suppressed. This results in any eventual residual production by the ovaries being completely shut off if the therapy is started during perimenopause.

You take a product similar to the pill; the packaging is identical. It contains 28 tablets for one month. For the first 14 days you take conjugated oestrogen, and for the following 14 days, you take gestagens. This is extremely important: if you still have your uterus, it's crucial that you take the combination product. Only then will you be protected against cervical cancer! There is a product on the market with a confusingly similar name that, however, is a pure oestrogen product. The manufacturer of this synthetic HRT specifies that the product must only be taken by postmenopausal women whose menopause took place at least 12 months ago — on average, 51-year-olds. Maybe this is the reason even conscientious doctors only recommend HRT to their patients when they have been experiencing symptoms for up to ten years.

The synthetic hormones are metabolised by the liver. This can lead to changes in the liver such as non-malignant adenomas (tumours). As the liver has no nerve pathways, it suffers in silence. Women with liver disease need to be careful here and possibly choose a different type of treatment. Other contraindicators are thrombophilia, hormone-dependent tumours, and clotting disorders such as an inherited factor V Leiden mutation. This is a gene mutation that affects the clotting system. The risk of thrombosis can, depending on whether one or both genes are affected, increase from ten to 50-fold. We mention this because approximately 8 per cent of the population has this mutation.

Caution is needed in women who are smokers or who have long periods of immobility such as long-distance flights or being confined to bed. Discuss this with your doctor.

Case study: An early HRT patient

Veronica, 74 years old, was one of the first women who had been able to experience sexual liberation thanks to the pill. Finally, she could decide when and whether she wanted to get pregnant. She chose not to have a family and to focus on her work. She had always reacted well to the pill and had been glad to have the option of moving directly on to a different hormone product after menopause to deal with the potential symptoms. Veronica had always been slim, she exercised, led a healthy life and never smoked. At the age of 66, she had a deep vein thrombosis in her leg as well as a pulmonary embolism, which fortunately was treated in time. The synthetic hormones were immediately stopped in hospital due to the thrombosis. After she left hospital, she experienced severe depression as well as anxiety, which she had never had before, and this resulted in her being admitted to a psychiatric unit. Four years later she was diagnosed with breast cancer, which was treated successfully.

In some women, stopping taking synthetic hormone products can lead to a genuine hormone withdrawal, with strong physical and mental symptoms. If the patient has been treated for years with substances that have a strong effect and a high concentration, and then stops taking them, it can have fatal consequences. Naturally we can't be certain whether there was a direct correlation between Veronica's sudden mental health problems and the discontinuation of synthetic hormones she had been taking for 35 years. However, considering the stable family situation and the lack of other risk factors, in my clinical assessment there was a clear link. Also, this patient showed no other risk factors (apart from her age) for a breast tumour.

Fortunately, synthetic hormones are now prescribed in low dosages, and there are also modern therapy options that we would now like to introduce:

New hormone replacement therapy with bioidentical hormones (BHT)

The need for an early and effective therapy to treat hormone-related symptoms in women has risen sharply over the past few years. And, of course, the therapy also needs to be safe: women want a treatment that allows them to take the lowest dosage of hormones possible and that is inherently more in tune with their bodies. Above all, a growing number of women want to address their symptoms during perimenopause more actively. We feel that this is a wonderful sign of women's increasing agency and empowerment. Why should we give away up to 15 years of our lives to a possibly unbearable situation, when we could do something about it? Why should we put up with side effects that could be avoided? Each one of us is as unique as their symptoms, and this is why a personalised, safe therapy is required, as opposed to an off-the-shelf, one-size-fits-some product.

Identical molecular structure

The desire to produce bioidentical active substances —i.e., those that are absolutely identical to the molecular structure as it appears in the human body — is not new. By the beginning of the 20th century, there were attempts to extract the corpus luteum hormone (progesterone) from animals. Because an extremely high number of follicles are needed, requiring a corresponding number of animals, this was not a feasible option. Another very cost-intensive attempt consisted of developing progesterone from its precursor, cholesterol. In the early 1940s, scientists were able to produce viable and cost-effective bioidentical hormones from raw plant material. In modern products this is diosgenin, made from wild yams.

The substance is also described as nature-ident, human-ident or body-ident. 'Ident' means 'absolutely similar'. In their chemical structure and their function, these products are actually 100 per cent identical to the hormones produced by our bodies. Within our metabolism, they behave like endogenous twins. But just as twins are two different people despite their similarities, so the raw material diosgenin is not an endogenous hormone. In order for it to be identically effective as a hormone, it needs to undergo further processes. It is only then that a pure bioidentical hormone comes about, and only in this way does the product achieve its reliable quality. But despite the additional processing, the raw material remains natural in its structure, and this also applies to its by-products. That is the crucial difference between these and the synthetic hormones.

We believe it is time to clarify the term 'bioidentical' and clearly and comprehensively explain which substances are used and what this means for your health.

In many online retail stores and, unfortunately, also in the research literature, the terms *bioidentical* and *hormone substance* are used for all sorts of things. For example, homeopathic substances are often extolled as bioidentical hormones, but they aren't. They cannot be used to carry out bioidentical hormone therapy, even if homeopathic remedies can help with symptoms during menopause.

It would be disastrous if a woman were to wrongly believe she was taking a bioidentical hormone in the form of the homeopathic remedy Sepia D4 and were to swap it for a synthetic hormone product because she wasn't seeing any improvement.

Even freely available yam root extract is *not* a bioidentical hormone, but a food supplement. Products available to purchase online containing pure diosgenin are not a hormone-effective product, whether in creams or mixed into yoghurt!

Application of bioidentical hormones

Bioidentical products for hormone therapy require a prescription, and the costs are covered by many private health insurance companies. Bioidentical hormones are currently the most popular form of hormone therapy among perimenopausal women.

Bioidentical oestrogen is particularly convenient, as it can be applied via the skin as gel (which contains 0.6 milligrams per gram of oestradiol) or as a plaster. In this way, the liver circulation is avoided completely, and the liver is spared. Also, the daily dosage can be adjusted individually. This is known as 'minimally effective dosage', which means that if hot flushes and exhaustion improve with two doses of gel per day, then you can reduce the dose to one a day and see how you get on with that. In this way you can work out your optimal dose. If symptoms of oestrogen deficiency develop, then you can quite simply increase the dose again. Hormone production in the ovaries varies a great deal, especially at the beginning of perimenopause, and you therefore don't need to replace precisely the same amounts of oestrogen each day or each week.

Hormone replacement does not necessarily have to be cyclical; it doesn't have to perfectly imitate the natural menstruation cycle. When you no longer need to use contraception, the trend is towards taking replacement hormones continuously, in order to better counterbalance the hormone system. This prevents fluctuations, so that the uterine lining is no longer built up and you no longer have periods. Without hormone replacement therapy, hormone levels continously decrease from around the age of 50. In HRT therapy with oestrogens, we aim to achieve hormone levels similar to those of fertile women at the beginning of their cycle. It doesn't benefit us at the end of our hormone production to reproduce the kind of fluctuations that only make sense in the fertile years. At this point, we need balance, not fluctuation.

We will now show you some examples of how bioidentical hormones can be applied in different hormone phases. Obviously, we can only demonstrate general and not individual recommendations — as always, it's essential to talk to your doctor.

Application during early perimenopause

SEB: 'Patients come to me with acute symptoms like hot flushes and strong mood swings or exhaustion. When I have ruled out all other possible causes and can ascribe the symptoms to perimenopause with an oestrogen deficiency, I recommend giving patients an initial higher dose at the beginning of HRT that will achieve high levels in the body straightaway. A practical start that usually works for most patients is, for example, three doses of oestrogen cream or gel per day. Cream or gel is applied over an extensive area on the inside of the arm. Anything from a few days to approximately three weeks later, the symptoms should have improved. If the patient has never used a hormone substitute before, then, after consultation with the doctor, the patient could reduce the oestrogen dosage. Depending on how well the symptoms are improving, they could reduce it to two doses or just one dose of cream or gel per day. If you already have several months of careful monitoring of your body's reaction to bioidentical hormones under your belt, then you can adapt the dose yourself. But I really only recommend this when you are completely sure.

'The dose adjustment applies exclusively to oestrogen!

Progesterone used as endometrial protection should never be reduced or discontinued if oestrogen is also used at the same time. Progesterone must always be taken as prescribed. If you experience excessive tiredness while taking progesterone, please talk to your doctor about reducing the dose.'

Bioidentical oestrogen products in gel or cream form are particularly suitable for reacting quickly to symptoms and for adjusting individual dosage. During perimenopause, hormone production in the ovaries fluctuates a lot — things no longer run smoothly. In one cycle there may not be enough of the hormone, in the next there might be the right amount or even too much. We can use individualised therapy, as we call it, to respond to these fluctuations. If, on the other hand, you take a contraceptive pill or capsules with the same amount of oestrogen each day in addition to the oestrogen that the ovaries may produce, then there is a danger of over-compensating and ending up with too much oestrogen. In contrast, after a period of acclimatisation, the individual dosage of oestrogen cream or gel is easy to manage if you listen to your inner doctor. Breast tenderness and water retention are signs that you have taken too high a dose. Hot flushes, 'empty bra cups', vaginal dryness, and mood swings such as tearfulness and irritability can be signs of a hormone deficiency.

Incidentally, hot flushes can also be due to a progesterone deficiency. At the beginning of perimenopause, when there is still a sufficient amount of oestrogen, this is often the cause.

If you are still having periods, even if they are irregular, with sufficient levels of oestrogen, then it can make sense to take bioidentical progesterone. We recommend taking two 100-milligram capsules of progesterone (so, a total of 200 milligrams) in the evenings. Progesterone is normally taken from the middle of the cycle onwards for two weeks — from day 14 to 28. Your period should start a few days later.

Application during perimenopause

If your periods are still more or less regular but you already have symptoms of oestrogen deficiency, such as dry mucous membranes, loss of libido, and irritability, then the oestrogen gel should be applied daily for three weeks. This application is known as cyclic application.

When you are undergoing hormone replacement therapy, regardless of whether it is with synthetic or bioidentical hormones, we recommend that you have all the regular routine gynaecological check-ups, including an ultrasound of the uterine lining.

THIS IS WHAT A TREATMENT PLAN COULD LOOK LIKE

The treatment period is 21 days up until the beginning of the treatment-free week, in which your period will begin. However, in a 28-day cycle, you don't start taking the dose from day one, but from day five. The first four days, meaning days one to four, are still considered part of your period, which is why the oestrogen hormone therapy is not started until day five. You then take the oestrogen from day five to day 25. In addition, it is extremely important for the protection of the uterus to take progesterone from day 14 to day 25, in order to prevent (oestrogen-induced) excessive growth. Please do not skip any days or reduce the dose! A dose of 200 milligrams of progesterone per day over 12 to 14 days will give adequate protection. The therapy then stops from day 26 to day 28, and so, together with the first to the fourth day, you will have a seven-day break during which you will have your period.

If the cycles become increasingly irregular, increasingly rare or you are no longer ovulating at all, then you can change the dosage to 100 milligrams of progesterone taken orally for 24 or 25 days. Then the therapy should be interrupted for four to five days. During this time, you may have a period, but not

---

necessarily. Following menopause, it is common to take the hormone consistently — in other words, without the seven-day break.

Application following menopause

One year after you had your last period, you would move from a cyclical or sequential therapy to a continuous therapy. No more support is likely to come from the ovaries, so now total commitment is required (if you decide on this option). In order to properly protect the uterine lining, you would need to take 100 milligrams of progesterone daily for 24 or 25 days each month.

Various forms of bioidentical hormones

How the various bioidentical hormone products are applied depends on the manufacturer and on your own needs. We would suggest that you go through your treatment options with your doctor in order to find the best solution for you. Naturally, your state of health, any pre-existing conditions, any chronic illnesses, whether you wish to have children, your general life situation, and family history including genetic predispositions, medication, and allergies all flow into the decision for or against hormone replacement therapy and subsequently, the decision about which product to take. Of course, your symptoms are the main focus, together with your wishes, expectations, and goals.

Bioidentical hormones are now available as ready-to-use products: oestrogen as a cream or gel that can be applied in a dose to suit the individual and progesterone in capsule form. There are also products that are prepared by specialist pharmacies (compounding pharmacies) after the patient's hormone status has been established. The dosage is adjusted according to the hormone levels. These products are usually taken in oil-capsule form. But let's take a look at the two hormone products separately.

Oestrogen

Bioidentical oestrogen comes in fat-filled capsules, called lozenges. These are placed in the mouth inside the cheek, where the lozenge is quickly absorbed by the mucous lining. There are also vaginal tablets where the oestrogen is absorbed through the vaginal mucus. In both types of application, the liver is bypassed. This is also the case for the most common type of application to the skin as a gel, cream, or plaster.

Some gels have to be applied over large areas; here it makes sense to use the thin skin inside the lower arm. Other creams only need a small application area. The difference is important for the effect and is often misunderstood. This is why it is very important to read the instructions that come with the product and to discuss the application method with your doctor. Only in approximately 5 per cent of patients is the gel not sufficiently absorbed due to the skin's thickness. If this is the case for you, try an oestrogen patch or other form of application. A hormone-level assessment should also be carried out to ensure that the product is having the desired effect.

Some women feel that their upper arms develop more cellulite when the gel is applied to this area for long periods of time. This could be the case, but in all likelihood, this is simply due to the fact that with increasing age our upper arms tend to store more fatty tissue and to lose elasticity. If you're worried about the gel causing wobbly upper arms, then you can choose the inner thigh or other parts of the body, like the shoulders, instead. Do not choose the chest area nor very small areas like the neck. In general, you should choose areas where the skin is thinner, because the ingredients can be better absorbed there.

If you get hot flushes at night and are starting to lose sleep, then it is a good idea to apply the gel in the evenings. This time also makes sense for many women who take the product in the evenings, because this is when they take the progesterone, which has a soporific effect.

Please note that you should not touch any other person (or pets) with the parts of your body to which you have just applied your gel. Otherwise there is a risk that you might pass oestrogen on to your family when you cuddle up together. And it makes no sense to apply your hormone gel before taking a shower and towelling yourself dry. *You* need the hormones, not your towel or your shirt.

Case study: Hormones are boosters!

Miriam, a 46-year-old photographer, had read up about hormone replacement therapy because of the psychological symptoms she was experiencing. She had always considered herself a creative and high-powered career woman whose job enabled her to travel the world and meet a lot of interesting people. For some time now, she had increasingly needed to rest, she found travelling hard, and she no longer enjoyed conversations with strangers. At times she suffered feelings of agoraphobia, and more and more often felt the need to withdraw. She described her situation like this: 'I'm feeling disillusioned and low, I'm sick of photography.' Ideally, she would have liked to escape to a remote island for the next few years. After other causes had been ruled out, it was clear that she was in the middle of perimenopause, confirmed by her barely detectable hormone levels. Her gynaecologist had already pre-scribed her oestrogen gel and she'd spread this on the inside of her lower arm without much effect. This is a phenomenon we often see. Especially at the beginning of the therapy it makes sense to rapidly increase the daily dose. Miriam, for example, needed three doses of oestrogen gel per day for several weeks until her lethargy and her depressive mood improved significantly. Her restlessness and free-floating anxiety also decreased significantly.

This patient's story shows how important the individualised and 'correct' application of bioidentical hormones is. Weeks of trying without the symptoms improving should make your doctor sit up and listen.

Progesterone

It is vital to take a sufficient amount of progesterone with oestrogen. This is the only way to prevent the uterine lining cells from growing and degenerating into cancer. The protection starts when there are 5 nanograms per millilitre (ng/mL) of progesterone in the blood, which can be achieved by taking one to two capsules per day. Earlier, we outlined the intake mode for those of you still having periods.

Caution: as mentioned before, if you are taking oestrogen, you must not stop taking progesterone without consulting your doctor — if you do so, you risk leaving your uterine lining insufficiently protected. Special progesterone capsules can also be inserted vaginally. This does spare the liver, but also means doing without the anxiolytic and calming effect of the progesterone. If you are not suffering from symptoms of anxiety, then the vaginal intake mode may have other advantages: the capsules help alleviate vaginal dryness because of their oily consistency, and you avoid a side effect (albeit a rare one): the hangover the next morning.

Time and again, the question of progesterone's efficacy as a gel or cream comes up, so we'd like to properly address this.

> SEB: 'In my experience, women with strong PMT as well as women at the beginning of perimenopause benefit from applying progesterone to the skin. However, this is only true for patients whose oestrogen levels are still in the normal range and who are not given *any* external oestrogen. With this form of application, the bioidentical progesterone stabilises the endogenous progesterone levels.'

If you do use progesterone creams, then regular ultrasound examinations are recommended to check the uterine lining. The data on protecting the uterine lining through progesterone is still inconclusive because the amount that is actually absorbed through the skin may vary depending on the skin's thickness. It is clear, however, that it is less readily absorbed through the skin than oestrogen is.

This is why you should only use progesterone creams if you are *not* taking oestrogen. For example, they may be appropriate if there is oestrogen dominance at the beginning of menopause, if the endogenous production of oestrogen is still sufficient, or in the case of larger women whose fatty tissue produces sufficient oestrogen. But only in those cases!

As we described in Chapter 2, progesterone calms the nerves and has an effect on many parts of the body. When it is metabolised, substances are created that have a positive effect on the brain and the nerves. Approximately half of all menopausal women experience some form of insomnia, and progesterone treatment can be extremely beneficial for this.

So, progesterone helps you to fall asleep faster and above all helps you sleep more deeply during the first half of the night. This is why it makes sense to take progesterone in the evenings and take advantage of its soporific side effects. Peripheral circulatory problems can also be a cause of poor sleep for people going through menopause. If the small blood vessels are not sufficiently dilated at night, the body temperature in the feet is lowered. This is why you may wake up if you don't sleep with a hot water bottle or woolly socks. Progesterone also helps with these circulation issues.

The calming and anxiety-relieving effect is mainly transmitted through the neuro-steroid metabolite of progesterone, allopregnanolone. This nerve agent seems to have an antidepressant effect and be effective against other mental disorders too.

For these calming effects, progesterone needs to be taken as a capsule or pill. Progesterone needs to pass through the liver in order for progesterone metabolites to be produced, which can then cross the blood–brain barrier. Those patients suffering from extreme anxiety can experiment with taking progesterone orally during the day, following consultation with their doctor.

Metabolic products of progesterone also dock onto nicotine receptors. In some small-scale American research studies, progesterone was found to reduce cravings for nicotine. Progesterone may therefore possibly reduce the craving for cigarettes.

Researchers are currently investigating neuro-steroids which are derived from progesterone for the treatment of depression, anxiety and other psychiatric disorders. The calming and anxiety-relieving effect of progesterone on the central nervous system is probably due to the fact that the receptors involved are the same ones which tranquillisers like diazepam (also known as Valium) dock onto. What is important in this context is that in contrast to the substance group of benzodiazepines (which includes diazepam), progesterone is not addictive.

When women suffer from depressive moods due to their declining hormone levels during menopause, it may be worth trying bioidentical progesterone instead of an antidepressant. However, it's essential that this is done in consultation with a mental health specialist, who can help you to assess whether your symptoms might be hormonal, situational, or connected with mental illness. Of course, one or a number of factors could be influencing your moods, so it's important to gain the assistance of a good psychologist.

How long should I be taking hormones?

There are different views on how long hormone replacement therapy should go on for. Some experts believe that, according to the current state of knowledge, hormone replacement therapy is safe for a period of around ten years. As nowadays hormones are prescribed along the lines of 'as little as possible and as much as necessary', this is a good position to take. We also recommend the strategy of the lowest effective dosage, as shown above. Preventative medicine today also follows a different approach. The assumption here is that the long-term consequences of low hormone levels only become apparent in the later years of life and that it is therefore sensible to treat classical diseases of old age such as dementia, osteo-porosis, and colon cancer with preventative hormone replacement. Supporters of long-term hormone intake believe that tissues and blood vessels in particular are protected well into old age. However, this only applies if hormone replacement therapy is started early enough. This thesis seems plausible, but further studies are needed to provide more information. Please discuss with your doctor, regu-larly, how long you should go on taking HRT.

Case study: An older patient with a rheumatic disorder and joint pain

SEB: 'The case of 65-year-old Yolanda powerfully describes how hormone therapy needs to be adapted to suit each individual. Her experiences really touched and surprised me from a medical perspective. Had I, for many years of my professional life, underestimated the hormonal aspects of the symptoms of older women without proven osteoporosis?

'Yolanda had been in treatment for her rheumatic disorder for many years as she was plagued by persistent, excruciating joint pains that often led to phases of complete immobility. Her muscles were tight, and getting up in the mornings was almost impossible. Although there was no definitive proof of a rheumatoid illness to be found in her blood tests or on her X-rays, she was treated as a patient suf-fering from a rheumatic disorder. She could only get through her day with the help of strong painkillers. For a while she was even treated with a very strong antirheumatic, for which we regularly needed to check her liver and kidney function.

'We now wanted to try a new approach, as despite regular visits to various specialists, a physiotherapist and spa treatments, Yolanda's symptoms did not really improve. Her hormone levels had fallen in line with her age, there were no signs of inflammation, all other blood tests were normal.

Although Yolanda was outside the therapeutic window of opportunity for HRT, we decided to try bioidentical hormones. The success was a surprise to us both. By her next visit to the clinic, she was no longer in pain.

'I recently ran into Yolanda. She walked over to me at a brisk pace and told me that she still couldn't believe that she was almost completely pain-free, no longer needed any pain relief, and was able to sleep properly once more.

'Of course, Yolanda has to have regular check-ups, and there is no guarantee that the long-term application of hormones at her age is safe. We talked about this at length before beginning her treatment. For Yolanda, the chance to get through the day without pain meant an immense improvement in her quality of life. She is more mobile now, and is altogether happier and more active. She watches her vitamin D levels, takes calcium, and has her bone density measured at regular intervals. Regular cardiovascular check-ups as well as cancer screenings (breast, intestine, and uterus) are extremely important.

'Fatty tissue produces oestrogen, so very slim people might need oestrogen supplementation (or, potentially, to gain weight). The risk of musculoskeletal disorders such as osteoporosis is higher for women with insufficient hormone levels. In Yolanda's case, she and I chose to treat her severe symptoms despite the possible risk the continued use of HRT might pose. Decisions like this are always tricky, and can only be done in careful consultation with a healthcare professional.'

In the long term, correcting a hormone deficiency in an age-appropriate and individualised way means preventing problems from developing later on. And it is only through good prevention that it is possible to provide for the best possible health and quality of life.

PHYTOESTROGENS AND OTHER MEASURES

Every symptom has its remedy — often in herb form. This is particularly true for menopause. If you take hormones, ask your doctor which phytoestrogens, that is, oestrogens from plant-based foods, you might take in addition. We now have good scientific evidence to prove that some of the substances found in nature have a therapeutic action. We would like to introduce you to the most important herbal remedies. Recommended quantities are only an approximate guide, as we do not know the extent of your specific symptoms. Please discuss the appropriate dose with an experienced herbalist or naturopath.

Oestrogen dominance at the beginning of perimenopause

Diindolylmethane (DIM)

A range of vegetables can help a lot. Many vegetables protect against cancer. Cruciferous vegetables such as broccoli, brussels sprouts, and cauliflower in particular contain the cancer-inhibiting plant colourant, chlorophyll, and diindolylmethane (DIM).

DIM is an antioxidant compound that is derived from the digestion of mustard oil (indole-3-carbinol). In 2004, an American breast cancer study showed that DIM protects against hormone-dependent forms of cancer by regulating the oestrogen balance. It can convert unfavourable oestrogens into favourable ones and counteract an oestrogen dominance. This also applies to environmental oestrogens in the body.

In order to benefit from the effect through food, the cruciferous vegetables need to be eaten raw. The content of the heat-sensitive mustard oil reduces by around half when cooked, and so does the amount of DIM.

> SEB: 'I have seen good results with the prescription of DIM, also in young women who were suffering from oestrogen dominance (swelling around the eyes or a general feeling of bloating due to increased fluid retention).'

What also helps:

- Reduce your alcohol intake. If your liver needs to worry about alcohol, then it will have less capacity to break down oestrogen. In other words: alcohol impedes the liver from performing its detoxification function.
- Eat lots of fibre, about 30 to 40 grams a day, increasing the amount slowly, otherwise your tummy will be rumbling a lot. Vegetables, fruit, whole grains, and linseeds are all high in fibre. The intestinal bacteria feed on fibre, which then helps the breakdown of oestrogen.
- Avoid 'foreign' oestrogens from the environment. Microplastic gets into our bodies via the food chain. A good start is to avoid drinking from plastic bottles and to buy unpackaged, unwrapped food, ideally organic, regional and seasonal.
- Eat as little animal protein as possible. Chose organic meat and milk products from cows who live free. Animals from factory farms are given hormones to gain more meat per animal, which means they are intentionally fattened up. The hormones end up inside those who eat the meat. Also, the use of antibiotics is common practice in factory farming; these enter the meat, and we then also take them in. This can cause antibiotic resistance to develop. If we should then require an antibiotic, it may not take effect. Antibiotics from meat damage our intestinal flora because this is made up of live flora. Last but not least, you'll be helping to reduce carbon emissions!
- Eat nutritious food and keep up a regular exercise practice to maintain your optimal weight. Oestrogen is produced in the fat cells, and when we have too much fat, this can result in oestrogen dominance. At least half an hour of exercise per day is recommended.
- Melatonin lowers oestrogen levels, and a product containing 0.3 to 1.3 milligrams in the evenings will also make you sleepy.

Treating oestrogen deficiency in perimenopause and menopause

Some plant ingredients exhibit structural similarities to oestrogen: isoflavones and lignans, for example. They have oestrogen-like effects and can be used to treat the symptoms of oestrogen deficiency. Studies show that these plant elements — called phytoestrogens — can significantly reduce hot flushes. However, we must have a healthy intestinal flora, because only then can herbal ingredients in the body have their oestrogen-like effect.

Soy products

In the 1980s, scientists from Europe found that not only certain forms of cancer but also chronic age-related illnesses occurred less frequently in Asia. The delicious, easily digestible traditional cuisine of Asia quickly became the focus of the research. In particular the daily consumption of soy products in Asia encouraged the scientists to take a closer look at soy protein. It is known that the phytoestrogens contained in soy products, the isoflavones, bind to oestrogen receptors and protect cells from excessive growth. The isoflavone derivative genistein also reduces those substances in the body that can cause inflammation.

Soy isoflavones can also counteract vascular changes. Eighty to 100 milligrams of isoflavone, taken in the evenings, improves sleep and also the blood circulation to the brain.

So, there is a lot to be said for soy. In the current guidelines published by the DGGG for the treatment of menopause — and likewise in other countries — soy products are recommended, particularly to treat hot flushes. Unfortunately, it is not enough to eat the occasional soy yoghurt or tofu burger; large amounts are required. There are a lot of genetically modified or pesticide-contaminated soy products on the market, so it's important to choose organic soy products.

Your body needs at least 30 to 60 milligrams of isoflavone per day. Some food supplements contain concentrated soy extract with more than 30 milligrams of isoflavones.

Red ginseng

This herb is native to China, Siberia, and Korea. The root, heated with hot steam and then dried, is used for medicinal purposes. Traditional Chinese medicine associates red ginseng with longevity and health. It is considered a general panacea. It does in fact help with many ailments during menopause, including hot flushes, fatigue, sleep disorders, and depressive moods. Red ginseng can be purchased in capsule form, but it is very expensive.

Hops

Regular beer consumption can not only give you a beer belly, but it can also give men beer breasts. No wonder, because hops contains phytoestrogens. In addition to the nutritional value, this was one of the reasons beer was traditionally brewed in monasteries: due to the high oestrogen levels, the monks lost their desire for 'carnal pleasure'.

Hops in capsule form can help with sleep disorders, restlessness, and anxiety. For women, hops strengthen hair and help with dry mucous membranes. However, you need to be patient, as the systemic effect only sets in after one or two months.

Valerian

Valerian has been used for centuries for anxiety, restlessness, and insomnia. If these symptoms occur in the case of oestrogen deficiency, we recommend taking valerian at night. Do not take it in the mornings or during the day, as it can affect the speed of your muscle reactions. Valerian can also cause headaches or gastrointestinal complaints. Valerian is taken in capsule form or as a tea.

Vitex agnus-castus

Vitex agnus-castus, also known as vitex, chaste tree, or monk's pepper, is a deciduous tree from the southern Mediterranean that has been used as a remedy for women's ailments for thousands of years. It has a stimulating effect on the pituitary gland and dopamine receptors. The release of LH is stimulated and promotes progesterone production. Vitex can regulate the female cycle and alleviate symptoms of PMT. It has a sleep-inducing effect and suppresses the appetite.

Since vitex counteracts a progesterone deficiency, it should be taken at the beginning of perimenopause. It is particularly suitable for mild to moderate menopausal symptoms. Women with very sensitive skin may develop a skin rash. You also need to be very patient with this herbal remedy, as it only starts to take effect after weeks or even months.

Black cohosh

Black cohosh is a perennial with white, elongated flowers, which is especially popular with bees and butterflies. As a remedy against menopausal symptoms, it can alleviate hot flushes and mood swings, and help with dry mucous membranes, particularly in the vaginal area.

For some women, black cohosh is the only thing they need to treat their symptoms; for others, it has no effect at all. The path through this phase of life is very individual.

St John's wort

The mood-lifting effect of St John's wort to treat mild depression is well documented. However, if your depression is severe, then you should see a doctor. St John's wort is not enough! It should also not be used in addition to pharmaceutical antidepressants. Liver values should also be checked regularly. Additionally, if you are still menstruating and taking the pill, then taking St John's wort is strongly advised against.

Maca

In recent years, this herb from South America has received a lot of attention as a superfood. In Peru it is considered an aphrodisiac. It increases the libido and general energy, and reduces stress. Maca can be helpful with treating concentration and sleep disorders, as well as hot flushes.

Linseed

Linseed contains the phytoestrogen lignans. What's more, linseed is a wonderful fibre. You can grind it up and put it in your smoothie or yoghurt. Once ground, though, it goes rancid quickly, and so should be stored in the freezer. Alternatively, you can grind the seeds in a spice grinder, blender, or mortar and pestle as needed.

Vitamin D

> SEB: 'I have been examining the benefits of Vitamin D for many years now. Fortunately, it has come to prominence in the last few years. I have never come across a patient in our European latitudes without a vitamin D deficiency who is not already taking it as a supplement in the form of capsules or drops. Some have a massive deficiency. The effects that vitamin D has on our bodies are numerous and the associated symptoms and clinical pictures are complex. I recommend most of my patients to take vitamin D all year round.'

Vitamin D modulates the immune system by influencing more than 200 genes. It has been proven that people with chronic vitamin D deficiency have an increased risk of autoimmune diseases, other chronic diseases, and some forms of cancer such as colon cancer (colorectal carcinoma). Studies have also shown that vitamin D deficiency raises the risk of type 2 diabetes. It can also lead to hair loss and mild depression: this is known as seasonal affective disorder (SAD).

Vitamin D is also essential for the health of our bones. The pro-hormone vitamin D controls calcium metabolism and promotes bone density. A sufficiently high level of vitamin D is vital, especially in the case of falling hormone levels that encourage bone demineralisation.

In 2019, researchers at the Medical University of Graz discovered a positive effect on blood sugar levels in a study funded by the Austrian Science Fund (FWF). In women with polycystic ovary syndrome, who also often suffer from insulin resistance, vitamin D had a positive effect on their blood sugar levels within a short period of time.

VITAMIN D: THE UNDERCOVER AGENT

The body can only produce 80 to 90 per cent of vitamin D as a prohormone if there is sufficient sun exposure to the skin. This means that the precursor of vitamin D is produced in the body. The problem is that in our latitudes — this would only change anywhere below the latitude of Rome — the sun never gets high enough in the sky in winter and we are dressed too warmly for our skin to make sufficient vitamin D. However, it wouldn't do us any good to run around naked in winter, either.

It is often said that sufficient amounts of vitamin D are stored for the winter months. But in order for something to be stored, it logically needs to be absorbed in sufficient quantities. However, due to very real skin cancer concerns, many people no longer go out without some form of sunscreen (many face creams and cosmetics contain an SPF 30+). Children are slathered in sunscreen and no longer go to the beach or into the water without full-body swim-suits. Many people nowadays don't spend much time outdoors, even in summer. They work in closed, air-conditioned rooms, travel by car or public transport, and then chill inside their own four walls. People who cover up their bodies and faces, and those with darker skin tones, need higher doses of vitamin D. This is why many of us need a vitamin D supplement to get us through the winter.

But what about the old days when vitamin D wasn't available as a product? In times before gaming, mobile phones, or working in front of a computer, many children and adults spent several hours a day out in the fresh air. During the winter months, we took cod liver oil, which is very high in vitamin D. Nowadays in winter, without sufficient sun exposure, cod liver oil or fatty fish on the menu several times a week, the vitamin D level drops by an average of 35 per cent.

The dosage of 400 IU (international units) of vitamin D per day as a supplement was recently doubled in the northern latitudes. The German Nutrition Society, DGE, now recommends 800 IU per day, but this amount is only enough to prevent an existing deficiency from worsening. If there are no contraindications such as renal insufficiency, a safe upper limit for adolescents and adults is 4,000 IU per day. You can find out the recommendations for your country online or talk to your doctor.

> SEB: 'I recommend my patients take 2,000 to 3,000 IU per day during the autumn and winter months, because most people's reserve has been exhausted by then and 800 IU does not compensate for the deficiency. It is important to determine the baseline value if the deficiency is to be followed by a high-dose saturation, and of course, regular blood checks need to be carried out. Over the last 15 years, during which I have worked intensively to address vitamin D deficiency, I am not aware of a single case of overdosing or any undesirable side effects. On the contrary: many patients are amazed and delighted with the rapid improvement of symptoms such as diffuse bone and muscle pain, tiredness, depressive moods, and a weakened immune system.'

The protective effect of vitamin D against osteoporosis has been proven. Studies examining its effect on autoimmune diseases and for cancer prevention are receiving a lot of attention at the moment. In the USA and Canada, vitamin D is added to milk, and in Great Britain, Australia, and Ireland, it is added to cereals and margarine (which we don't recommend due to the trans fats — see page 139 for more detail).

Important: We strongly urge you not to order high-dose vitamin D products on the internet. This can lead to incorrect dosages, confusing conversion factors, and incorrect types of vitamin D and its precursors being taken. In Germany, vitamin D products with more than 1,000 IU require a prescription. These recommendations are for healthy individuals. Caution is advised for those with kidney damage or other diseases, and we encourage you to consult with your doctor to find the level that's right for you.

> SEB: 'For people living in countries with year-round sunshine, the vitamin D values are above 60 ng/mL. So, don't get alarmed when people start to talk about the risk of overdosing. If we assess the various measurements and discussions and bring our own clinical experience into the equation, then a vitamin D level of 35 to 55 ng/mL seems to be beneficial to health and to prevent illness.'

WHEN IS HORMONE LEVEL MEASUREMENT A GOOD IDEA?

Time and again we are asked whether and when it makes sense to have your oestrogen and progesterone levels measured. Let's take a look at when it might make sense to measure hormone levels, and when it might not.

> SEB: 'When I left my gynaecologist's surgery in my early forties with my lab results, I was so shocked that I shed a few tears in my car. My oestrogen levels were at rock bottom, and the lab doctor had certified the low values as being *the beginning of menopause*. It was there in black and white, and I was devastated. When my hormone levels were measured again some time later, the value was around 100 times higher. How could that be?
>
> 'I discovered that this was a typical example of fluctuating hormone levels during these years. Whether the low levels were caused by a very stressful phase in my life, or whether I felt so exhausted because of the drop in oestrogen levels, I can't say with hindsight. The two are probably

mutually dependent. Despite the fact that I was still having periods, the ovarian control circuit began to stutter. This often happens from our mid-thirties onwards and shows that particularly at the beginning of perimenopause, hormone levels can stabilise again, and the ovaries can start working once more.

'In my case it was very helpful to see these values on paper, as they matched my changing moods. Patients are frequently told that there is no point in having their hormone levels tested because too many factors such as time of day, stress, different phases in the cycle, or certain foods would lead to constantly fluctuating results. I don't agree with this sweeping statement.'

For decades, the diagnosis of menopause was based on symptoms alone. As a result, it was treated with substances which physiologically do not occur in the body, and the need for these substances was never assessed using laboratory tests. Guiding symptoms can of course provide *indications* as to the underlying causes, but they do not provide conclusive *evidence* of hormonal involvement.

Today there is another approach to treating the individual symptoms. It's becoming common practice to measure hormone levels. An important argument for measuring hormone levels is to rule out other illnesses that cause similar symptoms, such as hypothyroidism. Night sweats, for example, can be caused by an inflammation or a chronic illness. It's essential to know the reason because completely different treatments may be needed.

The diagnosis of declining sex hormones is especially important for women who want to have children. If they are experiencing symptoms and their hormone levels are very low, it is imperative to establish whether the ovaries or the pituitary gland might be the trigger.

In principle, a doctor can work out, based on the hormone values, which phase of the hormone change a patient is in and how to best treat their symptoms. Measuring hormone levels may be useful, especially when symptoms start in your early forties or even in your late thirties. Then you have an initial value before starting a therapy and can be sure of what you are dealing with. This means you wouldn't take oestrogen if you already have an oestrogen dominance or be given progesterone-only therapy when it is oestrogen that you need. However, it's possible to test too often, and constantly retesting hormone levels would be just as ineffective as never testing them at all.

In the following sections, we will outline which additional measures can help you find your physical, mental, and emotional balance again. Our intestinal flora, the microbiome, is just as important as a healthy diet, exercise, a well-adjusted thyroid gland, and an effective way of dealing with stress.

Regulating hormones via the gut and nutrition

Our body can be compared to an exchange bureau. The currency is called food, and this is then converted into carbohydrates, fats, and proteins. Our food is divided up into these three units and is then available as energy. Given our busy lives, we keep spending our energy from our energy account, be it for processes in our cells, for the dash to the train, for a quick clean of our house, or for the struggle to come up with an excuse as to why we don't want to have coffee with that old friend. This is why we need energy that we can mobilise immediately to deal with the stuff that keeps us busy all day. At our disposal we have glycogen, the stored sugar from the liver and muscles. The term *storage sugar* is a bit misleading here, as glycogen is constantly being used up.

The *real* storage sugar is the other currency, our love handles, which we save for a rainy day. We are happy when we can go shopping, but we also make sure we have a nest egg. The need for security is something we have in our genes: put a little aside, you never know when you might need it. That's why every calorie that we don't use is stored on our hips and stomach for hard times. After all, for millennia it was common practice to fill one's belly when the apples were ripe on the tree or an animal was slaughtered, in order to survive for days or weeks afterwards. Slim people did not survive long periods of drought or bad harvests. Today the situation is reversed in many parts of the world: food is always available, and most people eat too much, too often, and burn fewer calories than they consume. As a result, they carry their ever-growing savings account around their stomach. This can cause health problems like high blood pressure, diabetes, and arteriosclerosis.

In contrast to sugar and fat, the body does not like to store protein. Proteins are, among other things, components of cell membranes and enzymes. If we eat too much protein, especially of animal origin, then there is an increased risk of colon cancer. So, the principle of metabolic control is therefore either 'Guys, energy over here, building material XY is missing!' to mobilise glycogen, fat, or some other reserve, or: 'What? Another delivery? We don't need anything now, off to the storage cupboard.' In this case, excess energy is stored as fat or misused for inflammation or cell growth. So, this is always the worse option.

What can we do? We can literally tell the metabolism to get a move on, through exercise (See page 154). And we can make our gut our ally by supporting it with more fibre and a fresh and healthy diet. What's more, we can watch our sugar intake and keep a check on our insulin levels. Along with the thyroid hormones, insulin is the hormone that intervenes the most in carbohydrate and fat metabolism. A low insulin level is a sign that blood sugar levels are stable. It is only then that body fat reserves are attacked — provided, however, that we do not allow ourselves to be terrorised by hunger. Hunger is the first to appear at the scene when the glycogen stores are empty. The first reaction is of course to reach for a snack. This is fine if it's morning or afternoon tea time, but if we snack too frequently, this can cause us trouble. Continuous eating, and thereby carbohydrate intake, leads to insulin resistance. This means that the body's natural inclination to burn its fat stores for energy will be weakened, as explained in Chapter 2.

Eating nutritiously dense meals, and not overeating, is our recommendation for a healthy metabolism and thus the best prerequisite for good hormone production. This is why we advocate a long-term change in diet rather than a crash diet in order to treat oestrogen dominance or hyperthyroidism. This way you counteract the yo-yo effect, and you don't need to worry about what's going to happen after your period of self-denial. You also positively affect the intestine. Not only is the intestine our largest organ alongside our skin, but also the largest hormonal gland.

THE POWER OF THE GUT IN REGULATING OUR HORMONES

More than 20 hormones are produced in the intestine, including the saturation hormone GLP-1, PYY, and cholecystokinin, the thyroid hormone T3, the stress hormones adrenaline and noradrenaline, and the sleep hormone melatonin.

Various hormones also coordinate the intestine's digestive processes, synchronise the metabolism, and influence the pancreas. Some of these hormones directly affect our behaviour.

New studies show that our intestinal flora uses the enzyme ß-glucuronidase to regulate our oestrogen levels. It is therefore assumed that poor gut health not only increases the risk of hormonally influenced diseases, but also influences hormone balance. And further to that: when we are brooding, angry, or stressed, our stomach does not just rumble for fun. It is actively involved in these feelings. We can often genuinely rely on our gut feeling.

Intestine to brain

Our stomach is rarely wrong. The intestine 'knows' more about our wellbeing than any other organ, even more than the heart or the skin. The intestine and brain are in permanent dialogue via the gut–brain axis, via nerve pathways, metabolic products, and hormones. We have 100 million nerve cells in the digestive tract alone. The gut provides the brain with a constant news feed: how much food is in the intestine, how long it will take to digest it, what's happening with the intestinal wall, are the intestinal muscles relaxed or not, and so on. The brain is informed and can evaluate what is important or what can be ignored. The intestine itself reacts not only to what is going on in its countless twists and turns or with the neighbours, for example in the kidneys, but unconsciously registers and reports on every stimulus in its surroundings. This information also rushes to the control centre in the brain and influences our thinking, feeling, and acting. The telecommunication service is managed primarily by the tenth cranial nerve, the vagus nerve. It controls the internal organs and functions like a data highway in both directions. Thoughts of someone special can cause 'butterflies in your stomach', while the memory of a recent fight with your friend can 'upset' your stomach.

However, our intestine also does what it wants. The nerve cells located in the intestinal wall are identical to those in the brain. They are not only anatomically identical, but they also use the same messenger substances (neurotransmitters) to communicate. This is probably why we sometimes feel our gut 'talking' to us even when our mind is still weighing up the pros and cons. Nowadays neuroscientists call this the *abdominal brain*.

A trillion little stars in our stomach

When you look at the abdominal brain, you can't avoid coming across the small residents of the intestine. For years now, the intestinal bacteria, also known as intestinal flora, microbiome, or microbiota, have been the focus of international science. We would not be able to survive without these 100 trillion bacteria, yeasts, and fungi. That's more little creatures than there are stars in our Milky Way. 'In fact, we are made up of 90 per cent bacteria and only 10 per cent human,' joked Andreas Stallmach, Director of the Clinic for Internal Medicine of the University Hospital Jena — and one of the leading microbiome researchers in the country — at the press conference of the German Society for Digestive and Metabolic Diseases (DGVS) in Berlin in 2019.

Indeed, our tenants control quite a lot without our knowledge: they fight toxins, split sugar molecules, and produce fatty acids, vitamins (B1, B2, B6, B12, K2, H), and amino acids. They ensure our intestine has an acidic pH value and thus prevent the colonisation of diarrhoeal agents such as salmonella. They regulate our cardiovascular system, our weight, our hormone regulatory circuits, and, above all, our immune system.

A healthy microbiome protects against chronic diseases such as diabetes, lipid metabolic disorder, and cancer, and, due to some new

131

studies, there is great hope that this might also apply to Parkinson's and Alzheimer's. Researchers at McMaster University in Hamilton, Ontario, Canada, are even convinced that the microbiome also influences our personality. They transferred the microbiome of confident mice to shy mice and, lo and behold, the shy mice were suddenly more daring.

The stress hormone level can be actively reduced not only via the vagus nerve, but also via messenger substances that the intestinal bacteria produce themselves. The intestinal bacteria are therefore also an indicator of stress. If everything is all right in the intestine, nobody is panicking, and everything is relaxed, then the intestinal bacteria tell the adrenal glands that cortisol production can be curbed.

French researchers were able to show that taking special intestinal bacteria (*Bifidobacterium longum* and *Lactobacillus helveticus*) for four weeks alleviates depression. The patients felt less depressed and angry, and physical symptoms were perceived to be more moderate. In another research group, *Lactobacillus casei* improved patients' moods after a three-week course.

But intestinal flora can do even more than that. In our intestine there is a bacterial species that stimulates our appetite. These bacteria produce the vital amino acids tyrosine and tryptophan, which are important for muscle-building, restorative sleep, and a balanced mood. A study has shown that eating a diet rich in tryptophan and carbohydrates has the power to reduce mental and physical PMT symptoms within just one day. Without fibre, tryptophan can stimulate excessive hunger and craving, so it's good to eat tryptophan in high-fibre foods like millet, oatmeal, or bran. This sends a calming, satiated message to the brain.

Our microbiome is sensitive and needs peace and quiet. Even if it does not really sleep at night, researchers from the Weizmann

Institute of Science in Israel found out in 2016 that the microbiome changes its activities at night. This day–night rhythm is dictated by our meals.

The intestinal flora gets out of sync through stress, shift work, jet lag, some medications, irregular food intake, and through a diet lacking in sufficient nutrition and fibre. We mentioned the health consequences earlier. Here are two more exciting bits of news:

Imbalanced bacterial strains in the gut, or a significant loss of bacteria (as with colonic irrigation or a course of antibiotics) can cause an undersupply or oversupply of free oestrogen. And a microbiome that changes with age can also damage the blood vessels. Until now, all we knew was that blood vessels grew stiffer with age. A new American study suggests that in old age intestinal bacteria produce molecules such as Trimethylamine N-oxide (TMAO), which promote arteriosclerosis.

Leaky gut syndrome — holes in the intestinal wall

If the intestinal flora is out of balance, undigested larger particles can adhere to the intestinal wall and cause inflammation and damage, resulting in leaky gut syndrome. This is where the intestinal mucous membrane displays gaps, particularly in the small intestine area. Leaky gut syndrome can be triggered by medication, stress, nicotine, pesticides, alcohol, and an unvaried diet. If the intestinal mucous lining doesn't seal properly, this can cause chronic inflammation throughout the body, as well as excess weight. The increased permeability of the intestinal wall negatively influences the insulin sensitivity of the cells, meaning that increased amounts of insulin are needed, which increases the risk of diabetes.

Because the intestinal wall houses more than 80 per cent of the body's immune cells in its mucous membrane, let's look more closely at this important natural body barrier. Bacteria and viruses that enter the body through food are intercepted here before they can enter the blood and lymphatic system. This is ingenious. This immunological defence is non-specific, meaning it works against everything. The immune defence cells (antibodies IgA) stage a targeted defence against unwanted bacteria; they appear in large clusters called Peyer plaques, in the mucous membrane. If an intruder has entered the body and caused trouble before, then the immune system recognises this immediately when it takes up contact again and launches the IgAs. So, an intact mucous membrane is immensely important for our immune system and also for our hormonal balance.

When we have a permeable intestinal wall, the amount of other bioavailable hormones in our blood is raised. This can upset the body's hormonal balance. In addition to an altered microbiome, increased values of the inflammation parameter zonulin can be detected, which is not only a marker for the permeability of the intestinal wall but is also connected to the reduced bacterial diversity in the intestine of PCOS patients.

So, there is a fascinating interaction between microbiome and sex hormones, immune system, and energy metabolism. This is why it is important to protect your intestinal mucous membrane with fibre-rich nutrition, stress reduction, and by not taking medication such as expectorants too often.

The microbiome — more is more

A species-rich microbiome is vital for our health. In other words, the more species of bacteria that romp around in our intestine, the healthier the person, and the more readily their body responds to exercise and nutritious food. Our intestine simply loves variety!

All the studies from the last few years prove this. If we review the medical background of some diseases like neurodermatitis or diabetes, then it becomes clear that the composition of the microbiome in these patients must have changed weeks or even years beforehand: the biodiversity is lower and so is the number of protective bacterial strains.

Scientists are now certain that many inflammations in the body originate in the intestine. If the microbiome is imbalanced, then the immune cells are not trained well enough — and in addition, the intestinal mucous membrane struggles with its role as a barrier. This causes bacterial components and other toxic substances to enter the bloodstream and lymphatic system, and to spread throughout the body. They can cause inflammation in the organs that are responsible for various cancers, especially in the digestive tract (liver, bile duct, pancreas, intestine).

Living intestinal bacteria, probiotics, have long been used to alleviate symptoms of chronic inflammatory bowel diseases such as Crohn's disease and ulcerative colitis. Now they are also conquering other areas: in 2016, Philip Strandwitz, from Northeastern University in Boston, discovered that there is a type of bacteria that survives in the intestine only in the presence of the brain messenger known as GABA. Studies are currently underway on therapy options with these special gut bacteria for depression, mood swings, and anxiety. In 2018, Aletta Kraneveld and her team from Utrecht University in the Netherlands demonstrated the correlation between certain types of mental illness and an imbalanced microbiome.

A combination of *Lactobacillus acidophilus* and *Bifidobacterium bifidum* improved the symptoms of depression in one particular study. *Lactobacillus helveticus* and *Bifidobacterium longum* also helped to treat depression when the patients' vitamin D levels were high enough, which raises the question of how probiotics might be used in the treatment of depression in the future.

HORMONE REGULATION VIA DIET

Our microbiome isn't alone in its love of fibre, wholegrain products, green vegetables, and fresh and varied food; our entire organism thrives on this kind of fuel. This applies to all phases of life, but especially to perimenopause. A fibre-rich diet prevents constipation, which can be exacerbated by oestrogen deficiency. It also makes sense to focus increasingly on foods with high antioxidant properties. They protect the cells from degeneration and therefore from cancer.

Fermented foods are a real superfood. They contain living bacteria and thereby contribute to the group of bacteria in our gut. The first person to demonstrate this was the Chinese microbiome researcher Liping Zhao. After he went to the US for a research assignment, where he ate a lot of fast food, he returned to China 30 kilograms heavier and with bad blood values. He then introduced traditional Chinese home recipes for weight loss into his diet, especially fermented bitter melon and Chinese yams. Over a period of two years, he lost 20 kilograms and his blood lipids also returned to the normal range. Because of the fermented foods, the composition of his intestinal flora had changed. He later confirmed his observations in mice.

We will now introduce you to fermented and other foods that can protect the body during perimenopause and help to regulate your weight.

Sourdough

Sourdough bread is in. That's good news for our intestine and subsequently for optimal hormone production through the intestinal bacteria. Like vinegar, sauerkraut, kefir, tofu, salami, pickled herring, and refined teas, whisky, beer, and wine, among other things, sourdough is a fermented food. The term *fermentation* describes the process of changes in a food due to bacterial, fungal or cell cultures. In ancient Egypt and Babylonia, yeast fungi were used for the production of beer and bread, and for centuries, vegetables and meat were also fermented. This was a healthy way to preserve foods without a fridge.

Because the fermentation process does not heat the raw materials, all the vitamins and other important ingredients remain in the product. In addition, probiotics are formed, which support the intestinal flora. These include lactobacilli, which strengthen the immune system and help to form essential vitamins like vitamin

C and B12. The fermentation process is also applied to the production of drugs such as insulin, hyaluronic acid, streptokinase, and penicillin.

Some foods ferment themselves — for example, black tea. Through the tight rolling in humid circumstances the plant cells in the leaves are squashed. As a result, air reaches the enzymes, phenols, and other ingredients and they react with the oxygen. Bacteria or fungi are added to other starting substances like hops (beer) or milk (yoghurt).

Fermented foods have an antioxidant, anti-inflammatory, and detoxifying effect. They lower cholesterol levels, promote the absorption of iron from food, prevent thrombosis, fill the stomach, stimulate digestion, and prevent flatulence. So, there are many good reasons to add a fermented product to as many meals as possible.

Fermented foods we recommend include: soy and yoghurt products, kombucha, kefir, sauerkraut, yoghurt, and kimchi. Kombucha is a carbonated, fermented green or black tea, which, along with healthy bacteria, also includes nutrients such as folic acid and iron. Kefir is rich in protein and is filling. In order for sauerkraut to develop its full potential, it has to be eaten raw. Sauerkraut is also rich in vitamin C, iron, folic acid, fibre, and lactic acid bacteria. Yoghurt with lactic acid bacteria should be eaten without any flavouring or sweeteners, as these undermine the good bacteria's work. For those with lactose intolerance, there is coconut, almond, or soy yoghurt.

Asian cuisine is rich in fermented ingredients: kimchi is a traditional Korean dish made from fermented Chinese cabbage, ginger, garlic, radish, and other vegetables. It contains fibre, vitamins A, B, and C, protein, amino acids, and minerals. Tempeh, from Indonesia, is made from fermented soybeans in roll or cube form and tastes slightly nutty. It contains all essential amino acids, proteins, magnesium, iron, phosphorus, and potassium. Miso, from Japan, is a paste made of fermented soybeans, which is used to make miso soup, among other things. Tofu from curdled soy milk is rich in iron, vitamin B6, calcium, and folic acid. And like all soy products, it contains phytoestrogens.

Getting lighter with fibre

Fibre is only digested in the large intestine, which is great, because high-fibre foods are the most important foodstuffs for our good gut bacteria. If the gut bacteria are sufficiently supplied with dietary fibre, they thank you in their own way: they prevent constipation. This can become a big issue during perimenopause, as declining oestrogen levels slow down the intestine's metabolic processes. Food then takes longer to be processed and eliminated. However, it does depend on what you eat. The less white flour and the more fibre, the lower the risk of suffering from constipation. Also, try reducing your consumption of animal protein from dairy products and meat, as they require more digestion and correspondingly remain in the intestine for longer. Fibre also helps to break down excess oestrogen and to get it out of the body.

High-fibre foods include pulses, linseed, spelt, oats, berries, dried fruits, nuts, and vegetables, especially cabbage and green vegetables.

Regular exercise also helps to prevent constipation, as do vegetable oils, magnesium, and drinking two to three litres of water per day. We recommend a tablespoon of olive oil with breakfast. Ayurveda, the Hindu system of medicine, recommends drinking a glass of warm water or ginger tea first thing on an empty stomach. This is an excellent, gentle way to wake up the digestive system at the start of the day.

SEB: 'While working on a book project on the microbiome, I changed two or three things in my diet. I now use oat milk in my coffee in the mornings, which gives me a good portion of fibre, and I no longer eat raw food in the evenings, such as salad, as this lodges heavily in the bowel overnight. I don't even nibble on a carrot stick anymore. After eating raw vegetables or a heavy pasta dish, I was sleeping badly — restlessly and too lightly — so now I have soup or something like that instead. I do actually sleep better. I have become very resourceful when it comes to making soups. It is surprisingly fast, too: chuck all the ingredients in a pot, add water or stock, season, puree, and you're done. I only allow myself something sweet at the weekends — I love every type of cake. In the past, I really needed something sweet in the afternoons — I thought I couldn't think straight without it. Once you have weaned your body off it, the sugar cravings reduce. This of course is very beneficial from the point of view of my altered calorific requirements from the age of forty onwards. And some foodstuffs I didn't used to like, such as olives and honey, now appear on my table.'

Tomatoes and unsaturated fats against cancer

According to the Adventist Health Study, run out of Loma Linda University in California, tomatoes protect against ovarian and prostate cancer. Unsaturated fats like those found in olive, canola, walnut, or flaxseed oil protect against breast cancer and other types of cancer, heart attacks, strokes, and diabetes. Eat plenty of them and avoid butter or margarine. The latter contains trans fats (hydrogenated fats), which consist of liquid oils modified for food processing. This makes the margarine spreadable, but trans fats increase the levels of LDL cholesterol and triglycerides, promote inflammatory processes in the body, cause insulin resistance, and increase the risk of heart and cardiovascular disease as well as certain types of cancer. This is why trans fats are prohibited in the USA, and Germany has upper limits in place.

Wonder weapon turmeric

Season with turmeric. Its active ingredient, curcumin, prevents inflammation and is therefore effective for joint inflammation and chronic inflammatory bowel disease. It also possibly inhibits the growth of cancer cells, especially in the intestine and prostate.

However, for this you need to eat large quantities (2 grams per day). We recommend one teaspoon of turmeric powered with a pinch of pepper — this promotes absorption.

> SEB: 'Initially, I ordered fresh turmeric from our greengrocer. Unfortunately, I really disliked the taste, and it also turned my fingers yellow for a week. I have since taken to drinking a glass of warm water with a teaspoon of turmeric powder together with ginger, a pinch of black pepper, and the juice of half a lemon. In winter I add star anise.'

Better without animal protein

Dairy cows are artificially inseminated in order to constantly be able to give milk. The pregnancy hormones from the cow also get into the milk, whether this is during conventional production or organic or pasture farming. Milk from sheep or goats also contains hormones, but often in far lower doses, as the production processes tend to be less intensive.

Alcohol isn't just fun

One for the road? Better not! For a long time, a glass of red wine every evening was considered healthy, but recent data suggests that even a little alcohol may be involved in the development of some forms of cancer.

Alcohol does actually provide some slight protection from cardiovascular disease, as grape skins contain the antioxidant resveratrol. Logically, this is also found in grapes. Also, alcohol is a real calorie bomb. And we would like to repeat once more: alcohol promotes oestrogen dominance and is a cell toxin, which, among other things, damages the thyroid cells. Our recommendation: drink alcohol in small quantities, consciously and with pleasure, eat red grapes and/or take resveratrol in capsule form, 400 milligrams per day.

Have a break

Of course, people have to eat. But not all the time. The body needs at least four hours between snacks or larger meals. Continuous snacking leads to insulin spikes, and can eventually lead to diabetes. Just as muscle mass declines with increasing age, so the fasting blood sugar level generally rises. The amount it rises by depends, of course, on eating habits, exercise, and lifestyle (stress, sleep).

Eat three large meals rather than ten small ones. And above all, eat regularly, because the microbiome also has a biorhythm. If breakfast or dinner keeps getting cancelled, it gets grumpy. It will definitely get grumpy if you are having hunger pangs at night, because it has other jobs to do at that time. Postponing your food intake because of shift work or jet lag, for example, is also not popular with the microbiome. It upsets the metabolic processes and leads to poor physical health.

We would like to address two types of fasting here — the 'fasting cure' and intermittent fasting. During the 'healing fast', the metabolism slows down and the basal metabolic rate decreases. The body empties its reserves (glycogen and fat), because its most important functions, such as heart, circulation, and brain processes, need to be maintained. Cell and DNA repair mechanisms start. The hormone regulatory circuits recover through fasting because the fat around the abdominal organs, in particular, melts, and its use as an oestrogen-production facility stops. However, fasting for a longer period of time should definitely take place only under the supervision of a doctor. Weight loss is not the main reason for therapeutic fasting — it's all about health. Often the two or three kilograms that are lost will be back on again, within a matter of weeks, as normal eating resumes.

Intermittent fasting, also known as interval fasting, is a healthy way to maintain your weight, and most importantly, it gives the body cells the time they need for repair processes. Permanently removing metabolic products from our food is pure stress for the cells and costs us a few years of our life. This is why interval fasting is considered to be life-extending.

When doing interval fasting, you have eight hours during the day to eat and then you stop eating for 16 hours. You can do this by shifting dinner and breakfast times. For example, you have your last meal of the day at 6.00 pm and then don't eat again until breakfast at 10.00 am. A coffee is permitted early in the morning.

WEIGHT REGULATION

Now we are approaching an issue that is hugely important to women. Particularly at the beginning of perimenopause, two-thirds of women are asking themselves how they suddenly gained so much weight. Those who are not happy about this often try not to eat any more than usual, or even try to eat less than usual, and exercise the same amount or even more — but they still don't lose weight. This can be very frustrating.

The well-intended advice from friends, doctors or diet books to 'just eat less and exercise more' is not helpful. Because it *definitely* isn't that simple. A two-week diet after which we were in shape again in our twenties now usually achieves a weight loss of only a few grams, if that.

Why do we put on weight in perimenopause?

There are several reasons for this. For one thing, the body needs energy for the monthly growth of the egg cell — ovulation — as well as the transformation of the follicle into the corpus luteum. From the age of 35 onwards, anovulatory cycles, where no ovulation occurs, become more frequent. Progesterone is partly responsible for the fact that the body temperature goes up by around 0.5 degrees in the second half of the cycle. If this temperature rise fails to take place, then the energy which is otherwise required for heat production is not used up. Even though many women don't notice the lack of ovulation, the energy consumption is nevertheless lower now. In the second half of the cycle, the body heats up seven degrees less, and therefore fewer calories are used up. After menopause, women burn about 300 fewer calories per day.

The other factor is that many women over 40 exercise less than they used to. Falling DHEA levels inhibit muscle build-up, and that is annoying because muscles are the best fat burner.

Resistance to leptin also often develops at this age. You constantly feel hungry. Physical activity is the best way to make the receptors responsive again, and thus reduce the hunger pangs over time. Exercise and careful eating help to reactivate the feeling of satiety.

As already described, oestrogen dominance leads to water retention and a redistribution of fat towards the abdominal area. The lack of progesterone affects the thyroid function and the thyroid can no longer control the oestrogen production.

Stress also leads to increased weight in a lot of people. We often see this in patients who are required to take cortisol products for long periods of time. Sugar in ready-made meals, the social expectation of alcohol consumption, environmental toxins, a predominantly sedentary job, not enough exercise — a lot of things might have crept into your lifestyle in recent years and might play a major role when it comes to weight gain.

If you are a larger woman, alongside the question of your hormones and whether you have an oestrogen dominance (possibly clarified by a test), you should also check whether you might have hypothyroidism, polycystic ovary syndrome (PCOS), insulin resistance, or diabetes. Is your microbiome healthy? A damaged intestinal flora after a course of antibiotics can scupper all your attempts at weight loss. Recent studies also found that toxins in the environment and in microplastics are being responsible for profound disturbances in our hormonal system. These endocrine disruptors interfere with the satiety hormone and the storage and the breaking down of fat cells.

WHAT DICTATES OUR WEIGHT

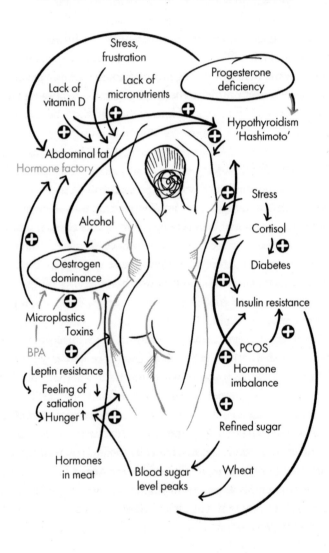

The good news is that up to 80 per cent of your weight can be influenced by your lifestyle. Thankfully, we are all now aware of the horrendous amounts of sugar in some sauces, fruit yoghurts, and other ready-made products.

> SEB: 'Although I have become much more careful about the food I eat, I am still constantly surprised, for example, by the fact that my favourite fig mustard consists of 89 per cent sugar. So, it is important to be on your guard and always read the nutritional labelling and know what's in the food you are eating.'

Stress-free weight loss

We deliberately don't recommend a regimented diet but argue for long-term dietary changes, and for moving towards a diet that mainly consists of fresh vegetables, fibre-rich produce, and calorie-free drinks such as water and tea. Everything in moderation — even a portion of chips with mayonnaise or a bar of chocolate, if need be. But not every day. It is worth addressing weight problems holistically: detoxify, reduce stress, change your diet, exercise regularly, sleep well and for long enough, and identify and treat hormonal imbalances. It is in the best interest of your mental and physical health that you try your very best to be kind to yourself. In a culture that equates beauty with youth and a slender physique, trying to love the gorgeous, perfectly natural body you have can feel very challenging. A well-loved body is a more relaxed body, and relaxation is crucial to health and to good decision-making (around food and exercise, for instance). Don't be too hard on yourself, don't set the bar too high. In your forties, you don't need to look like you did in your twenties or be as slim as your teenage daughter.

If you want to lose weight, it's likely that, at its simplest, you've eaten too many calories for your body to burn off. But *why* the calories were not burned off is a different matter entirely. Is it due to an illness like hyperthyroidism? Are you eating the same number of calories each day, even though from around the age of forty, your body cannot burn off as many calories because it has less muscle mass? Are you perhaps burning fewer calories because you move a lot less in your new job? Has your metabolism slowed because you are menopausal? These are all valid questions. The body cannot be pressed into a prefabricated mould, and your body won't react instantly or in the same way as your next door neighbour's body. Every woman is different, which is why the causes of weight gain are also individual.

A poor or overly rich diet as well as a lack of exercise are also part of the equation. Your genes are a factor, as is your hormone status, your age, stress levels, acidosis, toxins, and nutrient or vitamin deficiencies. Speaking of vitamin deficiency: recently, several studies have shown that a vitamin D deficiency can contribute to excess weight.

Eating can be a longing: the smell of a Sunday roast can remind us of our childhood; the smell of calamari reminds us of the peace and quiet of summer holidays, the crème brulée of a love affair in Paris. Eating can be social: the potato salad reminds us of our friends during our student days, the five-course meal of the festive and exuberant mood at our wedding. Eating can be a reward: a cheese platter with a glass of red wine sets the mood for the family dinner after a hard day's work: getting in, switching off, relaxing. Eating can also be affection: your partner surprises you with your favourite dish. Eating can be comfort: a bag of crisps or a tub of chocolate ice cream can help ease heartbreak and loneliness. Getting to know what it is you want to feel by eating whatever it is you crave can help you to start thinking about other, perhaps more satisfying ways to address that unmet desire.

Food diary

How am I supposed to know why I eat, and why is it important, you may ask? Try it! Keep a food diary for two weeks. It is fascinating to see what comes out of it. Above all, a good diary uncovers causes and effects and helps us to eat more consciously. You will recognise your patterns around when you reach for foods that don't really nourish you, or how many snacks you eat in-between meals.

What are your comfort treats? What do the different foods that you reach for represent? How is your mood when you eat? Make a note of your feelings when you eat your meal or your snack: how many calories do you need so that you feel full, or no longer feel stressed, angry or lonely? How often do you feel guilty, and when do you enjoy eating? Do you only eat alone and hold back in company (so that no one thinks you're greedy), or vice versa?

If you are able to identify the traps, then you'll be ready for the next stressful situation by bringing along a box of salad and a wholemeal roll, instead of having to resort to fast food or chocolate. If you manage to figure out your patterns, then you can teach your body that it doesn't need the stimulant *cappuccino with two sugars,* but that the relaxing *cup of green tea* would be a more deeply satisfying alternative. You have the opportunity to reprogram your brain.

Motivation is key

Why do you want to lose weight? Why forgo the delicious pasta and the glass of red wine in the evenings? It is not just a good question; it is the crucial question in order to maintain a balanced diet. Because honestly, why should you suffer without a good reason?

Why do you want to lose weight? Because it will lower your blood pressure and you will no longer feel dizzy? Because your blood sugar will normalise, and you will be able to do without your medication or reduce the dose? Because it will help you to feel better and more comfortable? Because you will be able to play sport again with your children or go jogging with your friend without getting out of breath?

Find the very best reason! Write it down on a sticky note and stick it on the bathroom mirror or on the fridge. Making uncomfortable changes is impossible without a good reason to motivate you.

Many studies show that social control increases your chances of being able to maintain your desired weight in the long term after a diet. Get your family and friends involved and allow them to rap you on the knuckles if you order fizzy drinks or junk food or want seconds just out of habit.

The journey is the reward

Don't be too impatient or too ambitious when you try to lose weight.

A scientifically proven realistic goal — and unlikely to result in a long-term yoyo effect — is to lose ten kilograms within 12 months (although, of course, this may well be too much for some people to lose). This rate of weight loss is healthy and can be measured in significantly lowered blood sugar, blood fat, and blood pressure values: for example, with a weight loss from 100 to 90 kilograms. A study conducted by the University of Massachusetts was able to show that diets containing less than 1,000 calories per day cause bad moods, concentration issues, and hunger attacks, and this then leads people to abandon their diets. So, please, don't torture yourself! That's certainly not in the best interest of your health.

Eat regularly, preferably always at the same times — even at the weekends. Then the body trusts in the fact that it will always be given good food and that it doesn't need to stock up in advance or go overboard later. This relaxes your brain; so, eating is not stressful, it's caring.

This is why you shouldn't skip meals. It might lead to quick short-term weight loss, but it's stressful and unsustainable.

Some artificial additives in food lead to a slight increase in weight, an increase in body fat, and elevated blood sugar levels. So, try to eat everything freshly prepared, if possible.

Vitamin D and weight regulation

The American Journal of Clinical Nutrition (AJCN) recently published a study showing that women who were given vitamin D as part of their weight-loss program lost more weight than those who did not take vitamin D.

The group who were given calcium and vitamin D as part of the diet also had lower blood pressure and reduced blood sugar and insulin levels, as well as low blood lipid levels. It was also shown that people from Asia were significantly more prone to obesity and insulin resistance if they had a vitamin D deficiency.

Scientists suspect that vitamin D sends out signals for fat burning, deciding whether fat will be burned to energy or not by directing special vitamin D receptors on the fat cells. If it is not used for energy, it is then stored on the hips. We recommend you have your vitamin D level assessed and, if necessary, rectify any deficiency.

Little stars in your tummy

A famous American study was the first to prove the importance of the intestinal flora to body weight: when the intestinal flora of overweight mice were transplanted into mice of a normal weight, these became overweight despite being on a diet. Swedish scientists proved that overweight people have less varied intestinal flora and also more bacteria that metabolise special carbohydrates in their intestine, which are in turn passed on to body fat cells.

We have since moved on a little further: we now know that a single species of intestinal bacteria can affect our weight. Overweight people often have less bacteria of the strain *Bacteroidetes* and more *Firmicutes*. Conversely, *Akkermansia muciniphila* protects from obesity. People of normal weight have 3 to 5 per cent of this bacteria in their intestinal flora, whereas overweight people have less.

The good news is that the composition of the intestinal flora can be actively controlled through food. Fermented foods, probiotics and prebiotics such as the high-fibre foods we mentioned earlier, ensure a balanced microbiome. With this good diet, the bacteria create their own metabolic products, including short-chain fatty acids with anti-inflammatory sugar compounds and substances that stabilise the intestinal tissue. This all helps to regulate weight.

In addition, complex sugar molecules, so-called lipopolysaccharides, are part of the cell wall of the gram-negative bacteria. In a sugar-rich diet, these bacteria multiply in the intestine and cause sugar to be stored in fat cells rather than burned. A very high-fat diet changes the composition of the microbiome; the intestinal mucous membrane becomes more permeable. Toxins get into the blood and can cause inflammatory reactions.

French scientists from the MICALIS Institute near Paris examined mice with a genetic defect for the hormone leptin. Leptin regulates appetite by passing on the information: 'Fat stores sufficiently filled.' It has also been observed in some overweight people that this feedback does not work sufficiently. These people are permanently hungry. Studies confirm the suspicion that certain intestinal-flora compositions may lead to better utilisation of food, and that in such environments, nutrients may be more easily stored than fat.

Why exercise is now non-negotiable

Exercise of any kind supports the metabolism and keeps insulin at a steady level. Our metabolism slows down from the age of 40, in particular because our muscle mass decreases. This causes our body to lose its best customer for the direct consumption of carbohydrates. You've probably been wondering why you need to exercise so much more than you used to, in order to maintain your weight. The reason is less muscle mass. Alongside endurance sports like jogging or cycling, we recommend a moderate session of muscle-building training two or three times a week. Make sure that the weights you are lifting are right for your body — discuss this with a fitness trainer. If you don't have access to a fitness trainer, a phone call to a gym will often result in someone kindly giving you a basic idea of the amount of weight you should be lifting.

Fallen off the wagon? Carry on as if nothing happened!

First: sometimes, it's so right to eat the muffin or the ice cream. Enjoy it! Second: if you find yourself eating in a way that doesn't feel mindful and supportive of your health, don't give up. It's normal to slip in and out of discipline. Try saying something kind and loving to yourself, and then returning to your nutrition program.

Third: it helps to set yourself a feel-good limit. At what point do you start to feel uncomfortable or angry with yourself, or for health reasons say: stop? This does not mean that you are weak or have failed. It is the same for everyone. Give an occasional dinner a miss, set yourself one or two diet days, or start taking regular exercise.

Hunger, appetite, or are you just not drinking enough?

When you think you are hungry, ask yourself if you really are. Hunger is often confused with thirst. Many people eat too much and drink too little. When you feel like you need a snack in-between meals, have a glass of water. Are you still hungry?

Do *not* go shopping when you are hungry. It's an age-old trick, but it still works: if you go shopping when you are hungry, you can bet on the fact that it's not just the things on the shopping list that will end up in your trolley, but also lots more sweet, salty, nutritionally poor foods.

If time permits, buy your food fresh each day. This way there is no risk of you eating up your supplies when you get the munchies. They will simply not be there.

Canadian researchers found out that eight hours of sleep promotes optimal weight regulation. Much less or more can lead to poor physical health. Those who have been getting too little sleep for several years have an almost 30 per cent higher risk of gaining five kilograms over six years. Leptin levels drop if you suffer from sleep deprivation. In addition, too much appetite-stimulating ghrelin is formed. Who hasn't experienced the munchies after a late-night party?

Early birds burn more calories. On average, late risers eat 250 calories more than those who wake up early. They also eat later in the evening, and have less time to exercise.

Changing your metabolism takes time

Have your scales remained unchanged for days now or you have actually put on weight? The first few kilograms of weight loss are usually just liquid that has been flushed out of your tissues, as the carbohydrate stores in the liver and muscles bind a lot of liquid. These are the first to be attacked when you go on a diet. Try to stay focused on your health improvement, and don't give much thought to whether you're experiencing significant changes in your weight and appearance or not, knowing that changing your metabolism in a sustainable way is complex and takes time. Fat is converted to muscle, and muscle is heavier than fat. Your weight is also subject to hormone releases, metabolic processes, etc. — all normal fluctuations. This is why experts advise against weighing yourself daily — once a week is enough. About one in five women have experienced an eating disorder at some point in their lives, and for many women, scales can be triggering. If this is the case for you, by all means, don't keep scales in the house. You can measure and track other (more important!) symptoms of a healthier diet: your mood, energy levels, and muscle strength. When you go the doctor for a check-up, this can be a good time to hop on the scales.

I have been invited out and I can't turn it down

Mentally prepare yourself for dietary traps like family gatherings, parties or birthdays, or work get-togethers. If you're at a buffet, it can be helpful to take a small plate. Avoid fatty sauces, choose fruit instead of dessert or cheese, and drink a maximum of one glass of alcohol. If all else fails, just go with the flow and pick up the healthy eating plan the next day.

A tip for former smokers

About 80 per cent of smokers who give up smoking gain around seven kilograms. It is likely that certain intestinal bacteria recover due to the absence of toxins and utilise the food better. The bacteria that recover are called *Proteobacteria* and *Bacteroidetes* and also *Firmicutes* and *Actinobacteria,* species that are abundant in overweight people. If you quit smoking and do not want to gain a lot of weight, then you should increase your intake of prebiotic foods and fibre.

And finally, the solution to a mystery

A banana contains as many calories as a bar of chocolate, but even eating five bananas won't make you fat. Why? Our intestinal bacteria gobble up the vegetable fatty acids in the banana, while the animal fats in the chocolate enter the body's fat cells. The solution, once again, is to eat lots of wholesome, energising, delicious fruit and vegetables. The more you do this, the more you will start associating fruit and vegetables with pleasure and feeling good.

Regulating hormones via exercise

As it is a well-known fact that exercise positively supports a diet and is also a 'miracle cure' for all other menopausal symptoms, we will now take a look at this subject. But don't panic — we're not expecting you to sign up for a marathon.

We would like to start this chapter with Alexandra's story, as this 'oh no!' moment seemed familiar to us:

Case study: Realising that your body has changed

40-year-old saleswoman Alexandra enters the changing room area of a large clothes shop. The obligatory mirrors line the entire wall on one side. As she passes by, Alexandra reflects on how vain society has become. As if the whole selfie mania wasn't enough. But hang on, who is that woman? She looks around but there is no one else there except her. Was it the light? She can hardly believe that the woman she sees reflected is herself. It's a shock because the body of the woman staring at her from the mirror is nothing like the way she believes her body looks. Yes, of course she had realised that she no longer had the body of a 30-year-old. But when had her body changed so much? Her breasts have become larger, her hips wider. She can't stop herself pinching the skin on her thighs — there was a time when she wouldn't have been able to do that. Oh dear. Frustrated and disappointed, she turns her back on the mirror. Strange, the last time she looked at the scales, her weight hadn't gone up that much ...

Many women in their forties have so much on their plate that they lose sight of their body for several years. They then 'suddenly' register the changes, as if their body had transformed overnight. Of course, that's not the case — the changes have happened gradually.

It usually starts with exercising less. Packing up your kit and getting yourself to the exercise class or gym takes time. Then you have to shower and drive home. You'd really rather save yourself that hour or two. You are already stressed enough, exhausted, you don't have as much energy. And at some point, you 'suddenly' find yourself in front of a full-length mirror, which you don't necessarily have at home, and you are shocked.

This not only affects your appearance. Abdominal fat in particular rapidly becomes a harmful hormone factory, promotes inflammations, and turns our hormone balance upside down. Weak muscles mean you tire more quickly and have fewer reserves. You get out of breath faster and are less motivated to challenge yourself. After all, everything is already exhausting as it is.

Less than half of German people aged 30 to 59 do no exercise at all. But in the case of women over 40, more than 70 per cent do no exercise — even though this is exactly the age when it would make most sense to slip back into your jogging shoes or your swimsuit. Exercise has been proven to protect against almost all symptoms that are associated with oestrogen deficiency during perimenopause. Regular exercise (or even just one hour of daily walking) reduces the risk of hot flushes, diffuse muscle pain, insomnia, and weight gain; it promotes bone formation and therefore helps prevent osteoporosis; and it protects against cardiovascular complaints and almost all cancers! It's especially important for women — regular exercise reduces the risk of breast cancer. Recent studies regarding leptin, the saturation hormone, are also interesting. The hormone goes off the rails in overweight people; exercise can restore leptin to the right level and thereby normalise the feeling of hunger, helping weight loss.

Exercise, endurance, and strength have ensured the survival of our species from the start. Prehistoric humans travelled more than 20 kilometres per day. If they couldn't run away from a sabre-toothed tiger fast enough and climb a tree, then they would quite probably be eaten before they had a chance to procreate. This is why our body is genetically calling out for exercise, because this ensures that all our metabolic processes are optimally stimulated, and every cell is oxygenated. Exercise builds up muscles, and these are the biggest consumers of calories alongside our brain.

Female muscles are generally smaller than male muscles, or let's say are 'narrower'. Testosterone, which builds and preserves muscles, decreases very slowly in most men as they age, which is why men keep their muscular physique for longer.

> SEB: 'I have a friend, an extremely wiry orthopaedic surgeon who, at the age of 55, is still running several marathons a year. He told me that the reason he exercises so much is that during his long career as a doctor, he realised that the musculoskeletal system is the factor that could most limit your quality of life.'

Many people can no longer exercise due to back pain and arthritis. Their pain hinders their mobility and restricts them in the same way women used to be forced into a corset. People with good torso stability have less back pain. One in three adults suffers from back pain often or permanently, according to the DAK Health Report in 2017. Menopausal women are clearly among them — they often experience diffuse back pain for the first time in their lives due to oestrogen deficiency.

> SKB: 'In my early forties, I had a back-pain episode in springtime for three years in a row. Despite physiotherapy, the pain lasted several weeks. As soon as I moved a flowerpot in the garden, got a chill on my back, sat for too long, or just moved in the wrong way, it started up again. I'm afraid I'm quite a lazy person but I had no choice but to lie down on my yoga mat and, after playing dead for five minutes, start doing the back exercises the physiotherapist had shown me. For this, I had to lie on my stomach and take turns lifting my right outstretched arm and my left outstretched leg several centimetres above the ground for at least ten seconds, or, even better, for 30. Then the other side. Ten rounds in total. Then the abdominals, because without an antagonist,

the back muscles have no support. In the beginning it was torture! But I have to admit, it was worth it.'

If you have good muscle tone, you will have a different body aware-ness and sense of wellbeing. On the other hand, those who don't do any exercise end up with a body that takes the view: 'What's the point of having muscles if I'm just going to lie in bed or spend the whole day on a chair behind the desk? I'll use the energy the muscles would have used to do the other things, so I don't need muscles anymore.' A study carried out by the University of Medicine in Copenhagen — albeit only on men — showed that after just two weeks of physical inactivity, the muscle mass in younger men up to the age of 30 had shrunk by a third, and in men over 60 by a quarter. It took more than six weeks to rebuild the lost muscle mass again.

After a week without exercise, you have probably been surprised to see that your jeans are looser around your thighs. This is usually not down to weight loss, but actually muscle loss. Muscle mass decreases continuously from the age of 30 by 5 per cent per year. So, at fifty, you have 10 per cent less muscle than when you were thirty. This is partly due to biological reasons — but only partly. Which leads us back to the lack of exercise.

Lack of exercise damages not only the muscles, but also the metabolism and the cardiovascular system, as well as many organs. Above all, the immune system is only just 'ticking over', which means that infections and fat cells increase. A vicious circle then ensues: more weight, less muscle. But every kilo you carry makes it more difficult to walk or chase after a tennis ball. Weight presses on your joints, and lack of exercise causes bone resorption. All the more reasons to stay seated on that chair you've been sitting on for eight hours in the office. It's not for nothing that sitting is now classed as the new smoking. That's how detrimental to health many experts consider lack of exercise to be.

Here is the fabulous list of benefits that exercise can bring you. There is nothing else that can literally 'move' so much at once:

- Exercise lowers the risk of cardiovascular disease, high blood pressure, high cholesterol, elevated blood sugar levels, arteriosclerosis, and strokes. Exercise protects against diabetes, because the sugar is removed from the blood into the muscle cells and burned there. This regulates insulin and prevents insulin resistance.
- Logically, exercise burns calories and, with sufficient exercise, also those calories stored as energy in the form of body-fat reserves: this has a slimming effect. The positive effect of exercise is felt even on a cellular level.
- Exercise is a stimulus for bone formation. Endurance and strength training are optimal for this — they maintain bone density, which can effectively prevent osteoporosis. As the muscles along the spine are strengthened, women who exercise regularly suffer less from back pain. The most important stabilisers for the back are the abdominal muscles. The better they are trained, the more support the back muscles get. You can imagine it like two weights that support one another. If you take one away, the other one collapses.
- There is synovial fluid in our joints that prevents the joints from rubbing against each other. This lubricant is like viscous oil. If it stands for too long, then it hardens. So, incorporate walking or bike riding into your life — your joints will love you for it.
- It is proven that regular exercise reduces the risk of colon and breast cancer. Even in people already suffering from these cancers, exercise improves quality of life and also improves the survival rate by up to 50 per cent.
- The brain uses more sugar than any other muscle in the body, and it is always glad of an extra portion of oxygen. Exercise improves concentration and memory as well as

powers of recollection and thinking. Exercise can help the notorious brain fog, that fuzzy feeling in the brain, to clear during perimenopause.

- Exercise can stop and even reverse inflammatory processes by means of messenger substances, whose concentration increases during physical exercise. Together with other proteins, these stimulate the formation of the small power plants, the mitochondria, in the cells, as well as many repair and growth processes.
- If you exercise regularly, then your body will draw on its fat stores and begin to break these down. Muscles form and tissues firm up. The scales might not necessarily show weight loss because muscles weigh more than fat. As we mentioned in the chapter about balancing weight: don't let this put you off.
- Another argument for exercising during menopause is the increased release of happiness hormones. You are more balanced, more satisfied, and readier to jump out of bed in the mornings. And exercise regulates your appetite.
- Last but not least, movement has been proven to delay the ageing process. Today we know that the inflammation parameters and cell breakdown are delayed by physical exercise. This is a wonderful concept: one lap around the park and you'll have one wrinkle less.

HORMONE YOGA

'Bringing body, mind, soul, and breath into harmony' — even reading this teaching from the old Indian philosophy can make you feel better. Yoga came to the western world at the beginning of the 20th century and is primarily practised here as a physical relaxation exercise. However, yoga is so much more than that: it brings people into harmony with themselves and their environment. Concentrating on one's own breath as well as doing meditative exercises lead to more calmness and balance.

The health benefits of yoga have long been proven: yoga strengthens the cardiovascular system, lowers blood pressure, activates the immune system, increases the ability to concentrate and harmonises mood swings. Postures (asanas), breathing exercises (pranayama), concentration (meditation), relaxation, and regeneration are the components of a yoga session.

Hormone yoga for women was developed by the Brazilian Dinah Rodrigues in 1992. The exercises are a mixture of classical yoga (Hatha yoga and Kundalini yoga), Tibetan energising techniques, and powerful breathing exercises. This combination specifically activates the female hormone glands as well as the thyroid gland and is suitable for women with PMT, those wishing to conceive and those going through a hormonal change. In Germany, the technique was further developed by the yoga teacher Claudia Lalleshvari Turske.

Through a special exercise in which breath is taken into the abdomen, thereby massaging and increasing blood supply to the pelvic organs, hormone yoga differs from other types of yoga. However, as with the classic forms of yoga, the holistic approach and stress reduction are at the forefront of this practice. This is because, as we will be showing, stress suppresses hormone production.

Hormone yoga moves the focus away from our mind or our thoughts, which are often the biggest stress factor. This is why one of the cornerstones of hormone yoga is targeted relaxation. This helps to prevent too much fluctuation in hormone production during perimenopause.

But you do have to keep at it and practise four to five days a week, or preferably daily, to achieve the full effect. The exercises will take around 30 minutes; doing them in the morning makes the most sense. Talk to your doctor before taking up hormone yoga if you suffer from hormone-related diseases, breast cancer, or hyperthyroidism, or if you are pregnant.

Four steps

In our experience, the right way to learn these special yoga exercises is by registering for a course, if there is one available near you. Even if you already practise yoga, hormone yoga is — in the positive sense — very special. Here is a short overview:

Warm-up exercises: before you start the actual hormone yoga, it is important to warm up and stretch the body. You can do the breathing exercises at the same time.

Pranayama: The breathing technique *Bhastrika* (bellows) and *Ujjayi*. For Bhastrika, when you inhale, the abdomen protrudes outwards like a pair of bellows. In the beginning, it is quite confusing. A tip: it helps to place your hand on your stomach and to breathe against your hand. When you exhale, you can trumpet like an elephant, as this allows you to best feel your breath. Before each exercise you should do these breaths five to ten times, in order to massage your ovaries.

For the glottis-breathing known as Ujjayi, you inhale and exhale through your nose with your mouth closed. The special thing about this breathing technique is that the air should whoosh through your throat with slight pressure. This feels as if you are trying to fog up a mirror with your breath — only with closed lips. This breathing exercise massages your thyroid gland.

Closure exercises: The closing exercises, *Bhandas,* control energy and keep it in the body. In the exercise *Mula Bandha,* you consciously close the lower pelvis by closing the perineum as if you were doing a pelvic floor exercise and maintaining this contraction for a few seconds. At the same time, you hold your breath and allow the tip of your tongue to rest on your upper palate. This sounds more difficult than it is — you quickly get used to it. It is an exercise that comes from Tibetan energy channels: it keeps the energy in the body. Then you focus your thoughts on the ovaries and thyroid and breathe slowly and consciously, imagining that you are breathing into these two organs.

161

Hormone yoga exercises: An exercise series might consist of *Adho Mukha Svanasana,* downward-facing dog, *Utkatasana,* chair pose, stretching the buttocks and hip muscles, *Setu Bandha Sarvangasana,* the shoulder bridge, and *Matsyasana,* the fish, where the head is arched right back with the crown touching the mat, while lying on one's back. The first two asanas activate the ovaries, the shoulder bridge is good for the thyroid gland and the pelvic floor, and the last exercise stimulates the thyroid.

SEX

Whether you sign up for a tantra course to learn what you most desire, or finally open up to your partner about how you might achieve a real orgasm, or whether you view your body as an erotic friend: let your imagination run riot. There are many ways you can have fun again. And you deserve it!

We would like to encourage you to give it a go, because sex and especially the female orgasm are in many ways the best medicine in a woman's life, whatever her age.

When the skin, breasts, vagina, etc. are stimulated, happiness hormones are released, the tissues are supplied with blood, and stress is reduced.

Have you ever noticed how smooth and rosy your complexion glows after an orgasm, how calmly you cope with the rest of the day: how patient you are in the long queue at the post office or when you're in a difficult meeting? There are many good reasons not to let sex wane, even, and in fact especially, if this simply means creating a self-pleasure practice.

Many women report that they have the best sex ever in their forties and fifties. By now you know your body, know what you want and what you no longer need. You have learned that you don't have to carry heavy emotional baggage through life with you — and that having sex for its own sake, without love, is a valid choice. Ideally, you express your wishes without feeling overly embarrassed.

You don't beat around the bush. Even though sexualisation on the internet has many downsides, and distorted, Photoshopped images of young girls can affect our notion of an ideal female body, the 21st century has given female sexuality a liberating push. Let's make the most of it, in the interests of our own health.

Sexologists from Vienna were able to prove that the level of the bonding hormone, oxytocin, is raised during orgasm. This causes the pelvic floor to contract and stimulates ovulation. When, by your late forties, ovulation is no longer an option, then bonding (whether that be with yourself or your partner) is the main benefit. This is why oxytocin, as we have already shown in Chapter 2, is known as the cuddling or bonding hormone.

Let's talk a little bit more about how this relates to single people, and to masturbation in general. When you orgasm, the happiness hormone, dopamine, is also released. This is similar to a drug as it activates the endorphin system and reduces pain. In addition, increased levels of prolactin are released. This ensures a feeling of satisfaction and also allows nerves in the brain to grow. Oxytocin, the love hormone, is also released, bringing about a feeling of loving and being loved, even if this is simply in a wonderful feedback loop with you and yours truly.

We have not forgotten that during menopause, many women's libido diminishes because of decreasing oestrogen levels. For many, sex is the last thing they want at that time. Often physical issues like vaginal dryness stand in the way of sexual pleasure. However, there are very good lubricants on the market, available from pharmacies and drug stores and even supermarkets. We recommend creams containing estriol, but check with your gynaecologist whether this will work for you.

Sadly, some women think that lust is something just for men. This is a problem that we will look at in more detail in Chapter 4.

You can have the physical wellbeing that comes from having an

The thyroid's role in hormonal regulation

It is not only the ovaries that at some point stop diligently producing hormones. As if the two of them had agreed on it, the thyroid also decides to take a break at exactly the same time — which is not ideal. This is known as the thyropause.

If symptoms of perimenopause or menopause such as night sweats and dry mucous membranes are ruling your life, then your oestrogen and progesterone levels need to be tested. Progesterone deficiency negatively influences thyroid metabolism, and then we have a serious problem. In many cases the symptoms of perimenopause and thyropause are similar, and are often confused for one another: 25 per cent of women in perimenopause also suffer from hypothyroidism.

If everything is lumped together, the symptoms cannot be clearly assigned, and in the worst case, they can be misinterpreted. If only the oestrogen or progesterone imbalance is addressed, and the thyroid hormone neglected, then the opportunity to treat hypothyroidism in a timely fashion is missed. Conversely, the symptoms caused by perimenopause require more than just thyroid hormones to treat them.

Thyroid diseases are often genetically determined. If you're concerned, ask your mother, sister, aunt, or grandmother whether they have had any thyroid problems. In chronic cases, individual factors such as stress, hormonal fluctuations, and infections can add up and, where there is a corresponding genetic disposition, cause the disease.

Thyroid disease impacts a lot of organs. The intestine and the thyroid gland, in particular, are connected. Thyroid dysfunctions and intestinal mucous membrane damage are linked. In the case of leaky gut syndrome, a different intestinal wall barrier disorder, or a disturbed microbiome, insufficient amounts of vitamins such as vitamin B12 or trace elements such as zinc and selenium are reabsorbed from food, thereby bypassing the thyroid gland. A recent study expressly points out that in the case of non-specific symptoms and either mild hypo- or hyperthyroidism, regular colorectal cancer screening may be useful, since both hypothyroidism and hyperthyroidism carry a moderately increased risk of colon cancer.

So, make sure that you have your thyroid levels checked during your next appointment.

T3, T4: OUR DRIVERS

Thyroid hormones convert food into energy in our body and thereby boost our metabolism. The most important drivers are T3 (Triiodothyronine) and T4 (Thyroxine). T4 is the inactive storage form that is converted in various organs such as the liver and intestine into the active T3 form. T4 is basically the hormonal raw material, formed up to 90 per cent by the thyroid cells. T3 is considered to be a biologically active thyroid hormone. It increases energy consumption, promotes the formation of the power plants in our cells, the mitochondria, and increases muscle mass. It also supports the formation of other hormones, including the happiness hormones dopamine and serotonin, as well as oestrogens, testosterone, and progesterone. Once again, we can see how everything is connected.

The trace element iodine is fundamental for the production of all thyroid hormones. It is not produced in the body itself; it must be supplied via food or air containing iodine. In the mountains, where the air is not so rich in iodine as by the sea, a goitre (struma), an enlarged thyroid gland, can take on huge proportions. Growth factors are released by the iodine deficiency, as the thyroid tissue tries desperately to enforce quantity rather than quality with the notion that more hormone can be produced through more tissue. In the past, it was more common to see goitres in people who lived in the mountains too. But we are now well protected by iodised table salt.

Every thyroid hormone consists of the amino acid tyrosine and one or more iodine molecules. The various thyroid hormones are numbered consecutively according to the number of iodine molecules they have: T3 has three iodine molecules and T4 has four. In order for T4 to become the active T3, an iodine molecule must be taken away. This requires an enzyme based on zinc and selenium. This is important as a treatment method.

Around 60 per cent of T3 is converted (from T4) in the liver, around 20 per cent in the intestine and the rest in the thyroid. This is another reason we need to be good to our microbiome.

THYROID
Where are the hormones activated?

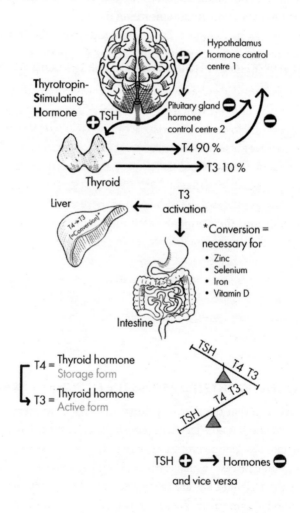

Hypothalamus
hormone control
centre 1

Thyrotropin-
Stimulating
Hormone

TSH

Pituitary gland
hormone
control centre 2

T4 90 %

T3 10 %

Thyroid

Liver

T4 → T3
(=Conversion)*

T3
activation

*Conversion =
necessary for
• Zinc
• Selenium
• Iron
• Vitamin D

Intestine

T4 = Thyroid hormone
Storage form

T3 = Thyroid hormone
Active form

TSH

T4 T3

TSH

T4 T3

TSH ⊕ → Hormones ⊖
and vice versa

You need to think carefully about giving yourself the best nourishment possible. Alcohol and a vitamin and nutrient deficiency can prevent the conversion of T4 to T3. Other inhibiting factors are stress, fasting, excess weight, medication, kidney or liver disease, pesticides, heavy-metal pollution, progesterone deficiency during menopause, and, unfortunately, ageing itself.

LESSER-KNOWN HORMONES OF THE THYROID GLAND

Alongside T3 and T4, the thyroid also produces the largely unknown hormones T1 and T2, which conventional pharmacotherapy has so far neglected. However, scientists are now paying greater attention to T2 than ever before. A 2015 study was able to demonstrate that T2 influences metabolism and body-heat balance. Additional research that will also look into weight loss, often a real challenge for patients with thyroid issues, will hopefully bring more clarity.

In addition, the hormone calcitonin, which has an important effect in calcium metabolism, is produced in special cells, and its antagonist, the parathyroid hormone, is produced in the parathyroid glands. Both are essential for bone metabolism. Calcitonin ensures strong bones. It lowers the calcium level in the blood by bringing calcium into the bone cells and promotes calcium excretion via the kidneys.

WHEN THE THYROID APPLIES THE EMERGENCY BRAKE

We have seen that the thyroid gland is involved in numerous bodily functions and has an effect on every single cell in the body.

In about 90 per cent of cases of hypothyroidism, the cause is an autoimmune disease, which leads to chronic inflammation, through which the thyroid cells are destroyed. The hormones escape into the bloodstream from these destroyed cells. They can cause symptoms of hyperfunction such as palpitations, agitation, panic attacks, sweating, shaking hands, and weight loss. With increasing destruction of the tissue, the focus will shift to hypofunction. No new hormone will be reproduced from the destroyed cells. Without the main hormone T3, all the symptoms of a reduced metabolism can arise. It can make you feel like the accelerator is broken, or as if you were going through life with the handbrake on:

- Chronic tiredness, loss of energy, low drive, debility
- Low moods or depression (the thyroid gland should always be checked in cases of depression)
- Weight gain, weight that isn't readily lost through diet or exercise
- Feeling the cold
- Joint and muscle ache
- Oedemas
- Diminished libido
- Inability to conceive
- Anxiety

A thyroid disease that is linked to hypofunction and that has reached almost epidemic levels in recent years is Hashimoto's thyroiditis. Seeing as a large number of women develop this particular form of thyroid disease, we will examine it more closely.

HASHIMOTO'S THYROIDITIS (HASHIMOTO'S DISEASE)

Hashimoto's disease is an autoimmune disease. This means that the body's defence system is compromised. It no longer knows who is friend and who is foe, and mistakenly turns on the body's own tissues. The cells of the thyroid gland are attacked, become inflamed, and eventually stop functioning.

Hashimoto's disease is the most common cause of hypothyroidism, and thyroid dysfunction is the second most common endocrine condition affecting women of reproductive age. It is assumed that one woman in ten will get Hashimoto's disease during her lifetime.

There is an increased risk during the phases of hormonal change such as puberty, pregnancy, and perimenopause.

However, the causes are manifold, including environmental influences. In Chapter 4 we will go into epigenetics (the external factors that can affect the disease's expression by up to 80 per cent) in much more detail. For now, we would like to point out that hormonal disrupters such as microplastics and plasticisers are suspected of inhibiting thyroid-hormone production and damaging thyroid tissue.

Hashimoto's can be caused by various chemicals and toxins, acute and chronic infections, the flu, and severe stress. Other triggers of the disease include food intolerances, like gluten or lactose intolerance (50 per cent of Hashimoto's-disease patients are sensitive to gluten), leaky gut syndrome, a deficiency of magnesium, iron, vitamin D, or some other nutrient, or a damaged microbiome, often caused by repeated antibiotic therapy.

Stress on a physical and emotional level (at times of upheaval such as divorce, bereavement, or bullying, but also due to shift work and chronic lack of sleep) leaves its mark. We don't want to be alarmist: not everyone who has stress will fall ill from an auto-immune disease. But taking care of yourself and making sure you factor in some rest is always a good decision for your health.

At the beginning of the autoimmune process, thyroid cells carrying hormones can be destroyed. If you could speak to your body, you'd say: 'Hang on, these are your friends!', but it would already be too late. Too much hormone is leaking from these cells into the blood-stream, and the damage is already done. Typical hyperfunction symptoms will become evident. When the destroyed cells are empty, then the process swings into hypofunction. With Hashimoto's disease in particular, so many different symptoms can arise, in addition to the hypofunction, that it's known as the 'chameleon of thyroid diseases'.

- Globus sensation, the feeling of a lump in the throat or pressure on the neck
- Oedema and swelling, especially on the face and extremities
- Frequent throat clearing and coughing
- Hoarse voice
- Dry, cracked skin, possibly itching
- Dry mucous membranes
- Brittle nails and hair
- Irritability
- Concentration disorders
- Nausea
- Digestive disorders
- Reduced libido
- Muscle pain and general weakness
- Stiff or swollen joints
- Carpal tunnel syndrome
- Neuropathic symptoms (formication, tingling, a burning sensation on the skin)

Diagnosis: better late than never, but ideally immediately

Because of the many faces the disease presents, Hashimoto's disease is unfortunately still recognised too rarely or too late. Many patients go to see their doctor because of exhaustion or depression, weight loss or hair loss. The most important thing is to simply be aware of Hashimoto's disease and to consider it as a possible cause of the symptoms.

Only extensive laboratory diagnostics can determine whether it is indeed autoimmune thyroiditis or whether there are other causes of the hypothyroidism. This is why doctors no longer only check the TSH (remember, that's the thyrotropin-stimulating hormone) value, but also T3 and T4, as well as the thyroid antibodies. In addition, an ultrasound of the thyroid gland is carried out. Of course, it is important at any age to recognise hypothyroidism as early as possible, but particularly in women who want to conceive. It can cause infertility, because low thyroid hormone levels could potentially disrupt the menstrual cycle.

SEB: 'Just measuring the TSH value can indeed indicate that something in the control circuit between the brain and the thyroid is not right, but it doesn't say anything about where the defect is. Therefore, it's definitely not enough to measure the TSH value alone. You also have to measure the antibody levels, especially in order to diagnose Hashimoto's disease, as this is an autoimmune disease. That is why TSH, free T2, free T4, and the thyroid antibodies TPO (thyroid peroxidase) and TG (thyroglobulin) need to be tested. The former is raised by up to 90 per cent in Hashimoto's, and the TG antibody by up to 70 per cent.'

The therapy

The active ingredient L-thyroxine (T4) is one of the most prescribed drugs in the world. Astonishingly, many affected people take it for years or even decades without their symptoms improving significantly. Paradoxically, the laboratory values often show something quite different: 'Thyroid hormones under L-thyroxine, all stable.'

The crux of the matter, despite lab test results being normal, is that the conversion of T4 into the active T3 form does not take place because it lacks the necessary enzymes. There can be many different causes for this disorder — chronic intestinal disease, microbial imbalance, selenium deficiency, and a liver disorder, to name just a few. The conversion or transformation disorder is often not recognised, especially if only the TSH value is measured to check the thyroid-hormone intake. This can turn out to be in the normal range, because the pituitary gland, as the superior hormonal gland, thinks everything is fine. According to the control loop, a release of TSH is not necessary if there is enough T4 in the bloodstream, and the drug L-thyroxine makes it look as though this is the case. Of course, the pituitary gland is wrong, because, as already mentioned, despite sufficient T4, the active T3 is missing.

The secret of good fine-tuning

This is why the fine-tuning of thyroid hormones is so tricky. If the symptoms don't improve, patients and therapists are often inclined to increase the dose of L-thyroxine. As we described in the section above, though, because of the conversion problems, this often achieves nothing.

Although T4 itself doesn't really have an effect, there is one exception: the receptors on the heart respond very well to T4. This is not necessarily advantageous. If L-thyroxine is the only medication prescribed during the fine-tuning of hypothyroidism, then this can cause heart issues such as palpitations, or even symptoms like those of an attack of angina (chest tightness). A feeling of anxiety or pressure on the chest is anything but pleasant.

Our advice: if you are having your thyroid tested, then you should know that the reference values have now changed. An upper limit of TSH was set many years ago with a value of between 4.5 mU/L to 5 mU/L. If you had a value of 8 mU/L, then you had hypofunction and L-thyroxin was prescribed. If the L-thyroxine value went down to 5 mU/L, then it was felt that the dose could be reduced. Today it is assumed that a value of 2 mU/L is optimal, as many women have severe symptoms even at a level of 4 mU/L.

There is no point having the lab results waved under your nose and being told 'everything's fine' if you are not feeling fine. Ask for the numbers, and if they aren't optimal according to your research, find a doctor who will take you seriously.

Here is an overview of the thyroid lab values to give you an idea. This may vary from lab to lab:

Thyroid value	Reference value (blood serum)
TSH-basal	0.27–4.0 mU/L Functional medicine recognises latent hypothyroidism from a value of 2.0
Free T3 (fT3)	2.0 — 4.4 pg/mL
Free T4 (fT4)	9.3 — 17 pg/mL
Inactive T3 (rT3) reverses T3	< 83 pg/mL
TPO-antibodies (TPO-AK, MAK)	< 35 U/mL
TG-antibodies (TAK)	< 72 U/mL

Adjuvant therapy with T3

Prescribing an additional T3 product can optimally fine-tune the thyroid. This is not always easy and requires a little patience.

Many doctors are either not aware of the possibility of treating a patient with T3 or they are very reluctant to do so. There are reasons for this: 30 years ago, T3 was used in healthy people to artificially increase the basal metabolic rate. It was thought that T3 was the ultimate aid to weight loss. But the medication significantly raised thyroid levels in people with healthy thyroid glands. This resulted in life-threatening complications such as cardiac arrhythmia and fever, and from then on, T3 had a bad reputation. This is unfortunate because when T3 is prescribed in moderation by a knowledgeable doctor to treat hypothyroidism, it can be a blessing.

SEB: 'I once experienced the negative feelings about T3 firsthand. A colleague of mine was outraged at the "doping method" I had prescribed. What was it all about? After a lengthy period of taking L-thyroxine, the health of one of her patients was not improving. Other physical causes were ruled out. Perplexed, the patient came to see me. Her T3 values were far too low — she was suffering from a conversion disorder, and the conversion from T4 to T3 was not occurring. When she began taking T3, reduced her dosage of

T4, and made some dietary and lifestyle changes, she felt like a new woman after just a few weeks.'

Reverse T3 (rT3)

Another player can also block T3: its twin, rT3, which opposes T3 by attaching itself to the same receptor and thereby blocking the effect of T3. It is therefore also worthwhile having your levels of rT3 checked: if your rT3 levels are too high while T3 levels are normal, then you probably feel tired and lethargic, which means that all the symptoms of hypofunction have increased.

You can lower your rT3 level by abstaining from alcohol and nicotine, detoxifying the liver, reducing stress, and taking a combination product of T4 and T3.

We would also like to mention an alternative to the conventional therapy with L-thyroxine.

Bioidentical thyroid hormones

Until synthetic thyroid hormones were introduced, hypothyroidism was treated with thyroid extracts made from bovine or porcine thyroid glands. The bioidentical version has been around for a long time, since the beginning of the 20th century.

Pig thyroid tissue is very similar to that of humans; alongside T4 and T3, it also contains T1 and T2, as well as components of the thyroid gland and its enzymes.

In the past, the amounts of hormones contained in the individual production cycles of a drug were inconsistent, as the extracts from young pigs showed higher concentrations than those from older animals. This problem is still partly evident today in the extract from cows, but basically the products are very reliable.

Some patients who struggle with the purely synthetic product can now benefit from the administration of the animal thyroid extract. They feel significantly better or are symptom-free. This may be an alternative option, especially for people in whom the standard therapy with synthetic L-thyroxine has not been successful.

In Germany, natural thyroid-gland extract can only be obtained through compounding pharmacies who produce individual medicines, and is only covered by private health insurers. Please check with your health providers for the situation in your country. These products are, of course, not suitable for vegetarians, vegans, or those whose religion does not allow partaking of animal products.

SEB: 'I have tried pretty much every option to treat my underactive thyroid. Of course, I started by taking L-thyroxine. However, my lab results as well as my state of health were anything but optimal. Whenever the T4 was meant to be increased, I suffered from an abnormally rapid heart rate. As the half-life of T4 is clearly significantly longer than that of T3, this is an unpleasant and long-lasting side effect. With additional active thyroid hormone (T3), the side-effects improved.

'Today I manage best with bioidentical thyroid extract from pig thyroid. Unfortunately, I have to order the drug in the US, pay for it myself, and when there are delivery problems, accept long waiting times. But it is worth it to me because with this drug I feel balanced, my metabolism is normal, I sleep well, and I am even-tempered. And my lab results are also good. I am not alone in this — a high percentage of patients in my practice claim that they were not fine-tuned when they were on purely T4 treatment.

'Even though I largely avoid meat products, I accept the compromise of taking a product that derives from pigs, for the sake of my health and wellbeing.'

Timing is everything

You can't just take your thyroid pill at any time of the day, though. Because it can interact with certain foods and other drugs, the absorption can be so reduced that you don't get the desired effect. This is why it's so important to take your thyroid medication in the mornings, at least half an hour before breakfast and away from other treatments. These include foods that are enriched with calcium, like milk and dairy products, but also orange juice, iron supplements, and coffee. Drugs that torpedo the effect of thyroid medication are cholesterol-reducing drugs, proton pumps, and acid inhibitors.

It can also be helpful to avoid food containing gluten and to top up your levels of iron, iodine, selenium, zinc, and vitamins B, C, D, and E if you are deficient in these.

Hashimoto's disease affects not only the thyroid gland but also the whole body, which is why we include in our treatment regime everything that strengthens the immune system. This includes stress reduction and, very importantly, liver detoxification, because only in an optimally functioning liver can sufficient T4 can be converted into T3. The adrenal glands are also happy and support the thyroid if they are taken care of. You can read more about what helps the liver and adrenal glands on page 183.

A well-adjusted progesterone level is important for optimal thyroid function. Progesterone sensitises the thyroid receptors in the tissues. The fact that thyroid dysfunction can be accompanied by hormonal fluctuations is unfortunately often neglected.

Supporters for the thyroid gland

Iodine: It is not usually necessary to stop using iodised salt when suffering from Hashimoto's disease, as iodine is extremely important for thyroid function, even if this is a point of contention. You should discuss whether the extra iodine is helpful with your doctor. Always pay attention to your body's reaction. Some patients need less thyroid hormone and feel more energetic during beach holidays due to the iodine contained in the sea air. Other patients complain of restlessness and other signs of hyperfunction when they eat various kinds of algae contained in some Asian meals.

Zinc: Zinc is a trace element that is involved in more than 300 metabolic processes. It is also indispensable for thyroid function because it is involved in the activation of T3. A zinc deficiency due to regular alcohol consumption weakens the immune system. Brittle fingernails, hair loss, and reduced fertility are just a few of the effects. Cashew nuts, almonds, seafood, sunflower seeds, and pepitas are rich in zinc. The recommended daily dose is 15 to 25 milligrams.

Selenium: Selenium lowers the amount of thyroid peroxidase (TPO) antibodies. It is important for the enzyme function of the thyroid gland and for the conversion into an active thyroid hormone. Selenium generally has anti-inflammatory properties and supports the immune system. In some places, including Australia and the UK, the soil is naturally low in selenium. This makes it all the more important to take in enough selenium through a balanced diet and, if necessary, to take it as a food supplement. Brazil nuts contain a lot of selenium; two nuts a day are enough to reach the recommended dose of 200 micrograms.

Vitamins: Vitamin B complex and vitamins C and D support the immune system. It's extremely important to have sufficiently high levels of vitamin D in perimenopause (see page 123 for more on this). This is why you should have your vitamin D levels tested if you have Hashimoto's disease and, if necessary, bring it back to the highest normal range.

Iron: A good iron supply is essential for the production of thyroid hormones and the effectiveness of enzymes. The extent to which a severe iron deficiency can lead to hypothyroidism is often underestimated. Have your iron levels tested and balance out any deficiency.

Balance out an oestrogen dominance

A progesterone gel applied directly to the area of skin over the thyroid gland can lead to a significant alleviation of the symptoms. If you've been paying attention you might be somewhat surprised because we specifically spoke against using progesterone gel in the section *Using our hormones to balance our hormones*. But we make an exception when it comes to the thyroid — try the application even if you have not previously taken any oestrogen. If you already take progesterone capsules, then in addition you can apply a small amount of cream to the thyroid gland.

Use less energy

The thyroid gland is the energy supplier for your 'home'. Not only is hypothyroidism often associated with persistent excess weight, but also more tissue needs to be supplied with energy. It is like a house: a large house requires more energy than a small hut. If by losing weight you no longer need to heat four rooms, but only two or three, then your thyroid gland will be happier.

Hashimoto's disease and gluten

It has been observed that the majority of Hashimoto patients do not tolerate gluten well, and suffer either from a gluten sensitivity or intolerance. In fact, antibodies against gluten can erroneously turn against the thyroid tissue, which is similar in structure. Gluten intolerance (coeliac disease) is genetically determined. Foods containing gluten like wheat, rye, and barley produce an immune reaction in the small intestine that can be accompanied by an inflammation of the mucous membranes. Those who have the disease experience abdominal pain with diarrhoea, weight loss, and signs of vitamin deficiency and fatigue, but anaemia, osteoporosis, and joint pain are also possible effects.

If you are not yet aware of a gluten intolerance but notice that your stomach regularly grumbles or cramps after you eat bread or pasta, then it is worthwhile self-testing for gluten sensitivity. Give up gluten completely for two to four weeks and see if you feel better.

SEB: 'Many of my patients feel better after a few days without pasta, bread, and those delicious baked goods made from wheat flour. Initially, you cannot imagine life without these things, but the adjustment is worth it. It will be easier to regulate your weight and digestion, and you will develop a whole new awareness of your body. There are many alternatives to bread and pasta. I have adjusted well to having an omelette or porridge for breakfast. Your blood-sugar level is more balanced, and you feel full for longer. This not only takes the pressure off insulin levels, adrenal glands, and thyroid, but also prevents hunger pangs.'

THIS IS WHAT YOUR TREATMENT PLAN FOR HASHIMOTO'S DISEASE COULD LOOK LIKE

- Rule out iodine deficiency
- Probiotics for intestinal health
- L-thyroxine with or without T3 or bioidentical thyroid extract in the mornings on an empty stomach, 30 minutes before breakfast
- 200 micrograms of selenium
- 25 milligrams of zinc
- Vitamin B complex
- Iron tablets if you are deficient (it is essential to take this at least four hours before your thyroid medication. Ideally you should take it together with vitamin C, after meals)
- Vitamin D 2,000 to 3,000 IU per day (please have your base value tested)
- Magnesium 200 to 400 milligrams per day (can have a laxative effect)

OUR HORMONES, OUR HEALTH

Last but not least, avoid stress. A high cortisol level blocks the progesterone receptors. If that happens our 'nerve balm', progesterone, has no chance of calming the system. We become charged up and jittery. The thyroid thinks there is already enough 'fire' in the system and curbs its production.

In the next section we will be showing you effective ways to deal with stress.

Regulating hormones via the adrenal glands, liver, and stress reduction

As we described in Chapter 2, the stress hormone cortisol is important in a situation of extreme stress or threat — in these instances, it focuses the body. To the body, stress always means you either fight, flee, freeze, or faun. Even if it's just someone tailgating you, or the telephone that keeps interrupting you just when you've sat down on your cushion to start meditating, this all signifies stress for the body.

Whether the horn sounds behind you or the doorbell sets your heart racing — we go into one of the above modes. We get nervous or aggressive; some people feel numb or depressed.

That is why the body *always* produces cortisol in moments of stress. It makes our heart race, our blood pressure and blood sugar shoot up, and we gasp for breath. At moments like this, our immune system is suppressed — there is no time for cell cleaning or any other detoxifying processes to take place in the body.

If the stressful time goes on for longer, say, several days, weeks, months or even years, then the body has a problem. It is more prone to illness, and it ages faster. Women who are exposed to extreme stress over many years before perimenopause age up to ten years faster than their more relaxed colleagues. This means that less privileged women are often in a worse position, as they may experience survival-based causes of stress on a daily basis.

A stress reaction is a remnant from archaic times. Thousands of years ago, when a mammoth had to be killed, for example, this was a hugely stressful situation. The animal was enormous, as was the danger, the weapons were modest, and the teamwork perhaps not great. But this mammoth stress probably only lasted a few hours; then you could live off the meat for months and put your feet up. That's if the findings from the stone age have been correctly interpreted. Today many people have to stifle their need even to go to the toilet, at least until their lunchbreak. It's hard to imagine!

Something is horribly wrong in our modern times.

In fact, most people between 35 and 55 are increasingly in a state of permanent sympatheticotonia, which means that the sympathetic nervous systems fire up all the organs to be in a permanent state of attack. This means the adrenal glands are barely able to keep up with the release of cortisol.

The antagonist of the sympathetic nervous system is the parasympathetic nervous system. It puts the body into a calming mode and ensures the functioning of all the organs that help the body, care for it, nurture it, and repair the cells. However, in times of stress, the parasympathetic nervous system is literally switched off. It can't get a word in edgewise, not even occasionally. But the parasympathetic nervous system would be extremely helpful at these times, as it's only when there's peace and quiet that all the players involved in the immune system can gather and fight external intruders like the next flu virus, or even cells that have run wild, such as cancer cells. But under stress, the immune system is suppressed. Many overworked people wonder why they get sick on the first or second day of their well-deserved holiday. It is very annoying, but not really surprising, because finally the cortisol system can be shut down and the long-suppressed immune system can report for duty with a sore throat, pointing out, 'I'm still around, you know.'

Particularly during perimenopause, women tend to be in the rush-hour phase of their lives. At this stage of life, it often feels as though a day would have to be 48 hours long in order to complete our to-do list. For those women who have children, they may be still small, which is exhausting — or they may be teenagers, which offers its own unique cluster of challenges. The double burden is extremely tricky, especially if you are trying to climb the ladder at work or if you are worried about keeping your job. Corporate restructuring measures have not decreased the workload. On the contrary, we have to do twice as much in the same amount of time.

Your circle of friends may also have grown steadily, and you don't want to turn down every invitation you get. Then there are the hobbies and other activities — both yours and, if you have them, your children's — plus visiting your extended family. Not to mention, you may have a partner who is still pursuing their career or already in the self-discovery mid life-crisis phase. You know what it's like.

During this hormone-rebalancing phase, we could certainly do without the stress, and most certainly the cortisol, which also robs us of our last remaining supplies of progesterone. Because this is what it does: as the adrenal glands produce higher amounts of cortisol than usual during chronic stress, progesterone is used as a precursor of cortisol. And that's not all, because cortisol is anything but a team player. Just like progesterone, it docks to the bone cells, and when the progesterone level in the blood is low, then cortisol can even cause damage: it stops the bone-protecting effect of progesterone. If, in chronic stress, too much cortisol is continuously applied to the bones, then the risk of osteoporosis increases.

It is logical that the adrenal glands will eventually have enough of this non-stop production. This condition is called adrenal exhaustion, or adrenal weakness.

It's worth taking a closer look

It is very important to recognise the onset of adrenal insufficiency in time to avoid falling into total exhaustion. People who want to please everyone and can never say *no* are highly susceptible to stress. Perfectionists are at particular risk. You can imagine how exhausting it is for yourself and others if you can never be satisfied with less than 100 per cent. Less is more here, and the same goes for the workload that some people squeeze into a single day.

Of course, there are external circumstances that we have already mentioned, such as the double whammy of raising children while holding down a job; an illness; bereavement; unemployment; existential fears, and so on, which massively drain your reserves.

You can never be on top of everything. But it is worth at least identifying the stressors — the triggers — that we can have some influence over. Often several stressors exacerbate each other, creating a cumulative effect.

We can say *no*. We can say no to a job that might bring more status or a little extra income, but which also brings three times as much stress. We can eat healthily, because fast food is stress for the body. We can ensure we have some relaxation and learn mindfulness methods. More on this later.

> SEB: 'The first thing you need to do is to realise that you are under stress. This might sound odd, but people often don't perceive stress as a problem. Stress has a very high addiction factor. The brain gets used to high levels of cortisol, and in a way, it seeks these cortisol-inducing experiences out.'

Human beings create situations that are familiar to them, even if they bring stress, or perhaps even *because* they bring stress. The reaction is familiar and, as we are creatures of habit, it is difficult for many people to say goodbye to stress. They would rather keep going. Also, chronically stressed people consume higher amounts of alcohol, drugs, and painkillers, and smoke more, in order to compensate for the consequences of stress. Unfortunately, that relaxing glass of red wine in the evening is not an optimal solution in the long run. You will fall asleep faster, but due to falling blood-sugar levels, you may wake more often during the night.

Due to a drastic increase in the incidence of exhaustion and burnout, and its associated sick leave and days off, there is more and more research into stress triggers and the physical consequences of stress. The findings have even led to a new branch of medicine: stress medicine. Research in this field is being conducted at full speed. Cynics would claim that economic reasons lie behind this, because people suffering from burnout tend to be absent from their jobs for at least six months. This is expensive for health insurance companies and employers. But we don't want to be cynical — so we choose to assume that it's instead about what's best for everyone.

Healthy cortisol release is subject to daily fluctuations. About an hour or two after getting up, high cortisol levels let us start our day feeling bright and dynamic. They decrease steadily throughout the day, and then a mini rise in the early afternoon gives us another boost. This is why we find it easier to step on the gas again about an hour after lunch. In the evenings, if all goes well, cortisol levels are back down, which makes us tired enough to sleep. Evolution knew what it was doing when it came up with this typical rhythm for human beings.

On the other hand, fluctuating cortisol levels due to sustained stress turn pretty much everything upside down: you can't get out of bed in the mornings, you drag yourself through the day — and the worst thing, when you finally can get to bed, is that you're not tired and end up tossing and turning all night. A living nightmare.

You can easily measure your own cortisol levels with a saliva test. This is a good and reliable stress marker. It reveals more about the condition of the adrenal glands than blood and urine tests do. Measuring cortisol saliva at different times of the day makes it easier to assess whether and to what extent the adrenal gland is affected. In order to carry out the test you need to give a spit sample into a small test-tube at three different times of the day and then send this off to a laboratory for testing.

A long-running chronic stress load creates elevated cortisol levels at the beginning of the day, and later, when the adrenal gland is increasingly exhausted, a decreased cortisol concentration in the saliva.

CHRONIC ADRENOCORTICAL INSUFFICIENCY

In conventional medicine there is often only 'healthy' or 'sick'. With regard to the adrenal gland, this means that it is either healthy, or largely no longer in working order. The latter state is symptomatic of a rare autoimmune disease, Addison's disease, where hormone production comes to an almost-complete standstill. Without hormone treatment, this condition is life-threatening.

But there are also the nuances: a weakness, malfunction, or dysregulation of the adrenal gland, called *hypoadrenia*. This is often not diagnosed, although it is common, and offers an opportunity to cope with stress in a preventative way.

An adrenal cortex exhaustion or weakness can lead to chronic fatigue and can weaken the immune system. Infections can become more frequent, and an autoimmune disease can develop, or another disease can become chronic. Also, cardiovascular disease, obesity, diabetes, back pain, and so on can be caused by stress; it can also cause brain dysfunction and a disturbance or imbalance in other hormone levels. If the chronic adrenocortical insufficiency is recognised in time, it is possible to counteract that slippery slope into burnout, or one of the many other diseases in which stress plays a part.

In functional medicine, a form of alternative medicine, preliminary stages of adrenal dysfunction are detected and treated. They are divided into three phases, from healthy to totally exhausted — that is, sick.

Questionnaire: how are your cortisol levels?

The following reasons or stresses can lead to adrenal exhaustion. You can expand the list with your own personal events that were particularly exhausting for you. A single extremely stressful or traumatic event can lead to chronic adrenocortical insufficiency, although usually the condition is the sum of several factors. If eight or more statements apply to you, then you may be susceptible to chronic adrenocortical insufficiency.

Physical symptoms

- I have had to take steroids (cortisone) for a lengthy period of time due to an autoimmune disease, asthma, or something similar.
- I suffer from a chronic disease like rheumatism, Hashimoto's disease, asthma, arthritis, or osteoporosis.
- I have been suffering more from allergies, asthma attacks, or infections recently.
- I have constant cravings for sweets or am hungry all the time.
- My heart is racing, or my blood pressure is rocketing without any external cause.
- I suffer from skin diseases such as eczema and my skin has become thinner.
- My waistline has expanded (circumference in women greater than 90 centimetres, BMI higher than 25).
- My blood sugar is unbalanced and often fluctuates. It may be elevated, or prediabetes may have been diagnosed. Or a state of hypoglycaemia may have occurred with trembling, sweating, agitation, and aggressiveness.
- I suffer from insulin resistance.
- I suffer from gastrointestinal problems or heartburn.
- My periods have become irregular.
- I am increasingly sensitive to cold and need socks in bed at night.
- The skin on the inside of my lips and on my nipples and vulva has turned significantly darker than it used to be.
- Brown spots have appeared on my shoulders, neck, and face.
- I have a muscle weakness.
- My eyelids are swollen in the morning, my ankles in the evening.
- I wake up in the morning, or between 1.00 am and 4.00 am during the night, with anxiety and palpitations, often due to nightmares.

Mental issues

- I have had extremely stressful phases over the last few years (separation, divorce, moving to a new house, changing jobs, caring for relatives, bereavement, conflict at work, unemployment, existential fears). These have brought me to the edge of exhaustion.
- I am not as productive in my job, nor as resilient or as efficient as I used to be.
- I have trouble concentrating and struggle to find the words I'm looking for.
- I flip out quickly, get angry very quickly, and am easily annoyed.
- I suffer from emotional ups and downs, and am often sad.
- I rush from one thing to the next all day long.
- I am anxious and constantly worry about things.
- My relationships — including with friends — have become problematic. There has been a lot of conflict recently.
- I keep meaning to take some time out and find some peace and quiet, but I never manage to.
- I constantly feel the urge to lie down.
- I have become more sensitive to noise and am easily startled.
- My libido has diminished.
- I feel listless, without hope, desperate, and weak.
- I feel much less joy than I used to, and everything feels like a burden.

Typically changed biorhythm and eating patterns in chronic adrenocortical insufficiency

Between 7.00 am and 9.00 am, you just don't want to get out of bed, and it's generally hard to get up in the mornings. It's easily 10.00 am by the time you are properly awake; you've had at least two cups of coffee by this point.

By 3.00 pm your energy has plummeted, and you have to drag your way through the afternoon if you don't have even more coffee.

By 9.00 pm you are so tired that you have to make a real effort not to fall asleep. However, you should not wait too long to do so, because if you miss the window of opportunity, then there will be a surge of energy around 11.00 pm, resulting in feeling tired and wired. You lie awake and can't sleep. Now you should pick up a good book or magazine instead of scrolling on your tablet or watching a film on television. Otherwise, the light source will cause the sleep hormone melatonin to be suppressed, and the body will think that it's time to get up at around midnight.

Fasting in any form is difficult, even intermittent fasting. The addiction to sweets, even to fruit because of the fruit sugar, is strong. At times of stress in particular, you may eat at irregular times and you end up eating too much.

Therapy for chronic adrenocortical insufficiency (CAI)

Bedtime treat: Although we generally don't recommend late meals or snacks, eating something low in sugar and carbohydrates and high in protein, such as plain yoghurt, just before you go to bed can be helpful if you have chronic adrenocortical insufficiency, in order to avoid waking up at night. But try to make sure you eat your last big meal before 6.00 pm and preferably include plenty of fibre. Your blood sugar rises rapidly and then rushes down again when you consume products containing fast-acting refined carbohydrates, such as white bread or pasta, causing you to wake up during the night.

Not too much fructose: Do not eat too much fruit, especially in the mornings. The fruit sugar content increases blood sugar levels too fast. Insulin levels shoot up and clear all the sugar out of your bloodstream, which can result in hypoglycaemia. This can cause some women to feel shaky after breakfast.

A pinch of salt: Use the saltshaker: people with adrenal insufficiency often have low blood pressure. So, if you have CAI, you might need to be more generous with the salt. Use Himalayan salt, organic sea salt, or algae products. Good sources of salt include olives, seaweed, spinach, celery, and zucchini.

Eat wholefoods: Your food should be rich in vitamins and minerals; empty storage cells worsen the exhaustion. Following many years of a vegetarian or vegan diet, vitamin B12 is often lacking, so it's a good idea to take a supplement.

Sex: We would like to encourage you to have sex. It will not only to help you fall asleep, but it acts as a natural remedy to stress. Make the most of it: an orgasm relaxes you and floods the body with oxytocin.

Sleeping on prescription: Those of us who are parents try to make sure that our children get enough sleep, but we often don't do the same for ourselves. If you feel exhausted, then sleep is the be-all and end-all and not a weakness. Choosing to go to bed early because you're tired does not make you boring and is not something to be ashamed of. Those who boast that they only need four hours of sleep are, to say the least, not a healthy role model — they will age faster and put themselves at risk of disease.

Night-time is when all the repair mechanisms take place in our cells, including the adrenal cells. So, sleep is the best prevention!

Late risers preferred: If you have CAI and your work or daily life allows it, you should stay in bed until 9.00 am or even 10.00 am. If this is not possible during the week, then at least do this at the weekends. This is the time of day when cortisol is at its highest. When the body demands high cortisol levels for a long period of time, then at some point the adrenal glands go on strike and produce less of it, resulting in a morning low. If you are permanently fighting this, then it will worsen the CAI. Your adrenal glands, or rather your whole body, now needs exactly the opposite: recovery instead of even more stress. If you struggle to get up, then stay lying down and please don't feel guilty about it. You can sleep until 9.00 am on doctor's orders!

Adaptogens for the adrenal gland: Adaptogens are plant substances that support the body in dealing with stress. In other words, they increase our resistance to stress. They come in capsule or tablet form, as a food supplement, and as a tea, and you can find them in the organic food section even in some supermarkets. These products have few side effects and can usually be taken daily, but pay attention to the information on the pack.

Roseroot is a plant that can withstand very cold temperatures. It has been shown to reduce the release of cortisol and thus arms the body against stress. Roseroot is also said to delay skin ageing and the formation of wrinkles.

Siberian ginseng is used as a power root in traditional Chinese medicine. It has a performance-enhancing effect, increases stress resistance, activates the metabolism, acts as an anxiolytic, relieves anxiety, is an antidepressant, improves sleep, normalises blood sugars, and makes you happy because it promotes the production of the happiness hormones serotonin and dopamine.

Vitamin C catches free radicals, which are created as cell waste products and weaken the immune system. This vitamin is involved in the formation of hormones, the absorption of iron in the intestines and the blocking of carcinogenic nitrogen compounds (nitrosamines).

Shiitake mushrooms act against stress, strengthen the immune system as well as the microbiome, and have positive effects on blood lipids.

Ashwagandha, or *Sleeping berry,* as this fruit is popularly known, calms the mind and has a balancing effect on the body. This is why it is a natural sleep aid.

Ginger normalises blood pressure and heart rate and stimulates the digestion.

Ginkgo biloba extract stems from one of the oldest tree species in the world. It is known to enhance circulation in the brain's blood vessels. Ginkgo is also said to protect our cells from free radicals.

Adrenal extracts: Adrenal extracts provide precursors and building blocks for hormone production and are possibly also small hormone doses themselves. They are important for restoring adrenal function. The idea is to help people to help themselves.

It is known that the destruction of the adrenal gland, for example after severe influenza, is not caused only by the infection, but also by exhaustion. Many patients used to benefit from adrenal extracts from bovine adrenal glands until synthetic glucocorticoids became available. Today natural adrenal extracts to get you back on your feet faster can be ordered over the counter from pharmacies. If this is suitable for you, discuss this option with your doctor.

Avoid caffeine. There is nothing better than a delicious coffee, but in times of stress, caffeine does not provide energy — in fact, it takes it away from us:

Coffee has been hyped for years. Coffee can reduce the risk of strokes and Alzheimer's disease and is supposed to have liver-protecting properties. So, coffee is a very worthwhile drink.

However, in stressful times, coffee can also lead to a deterioration in the state of your health. From four or five cups a day upwards, coffee can become toxic and change your sleep rhythm. Coffee also raises the levels of cortisol and insulin. This leads to a merciless storage of fat, turns the circadian rhythm upside down, and works against hormonal balance. Make sure that you don't get into that vicious cycle: stress-overtiredness-coffee-nervousness-sleep, or, disorder-fatigue-coffee. You might have observed that after a coffee, you feel nervous or exhilarated, and then soon after that, irritable. This is a sign that you might be happier and healthier without it.

Caffeine can block control loops in the body that calm our

system. Typically, as a reaction to coffee, people suffering from CAI can experience sudden tiredness; you can then fall into a hole, followed by a craving for sweets, in order to revive the circulation.

Count how many cups you drink in a day. Caffeine is addictive; it increases our dopamine production and thus leads to dependency.

Decaffeinated coffee is unfortunately only half the solution. Through its acids, it also has an influence on blood sugar, cortisol, and the activity of the sympathetic nervous system. You'll remember: flight or fight.

In CAI, it is important to limit coffee consumption to a maximum of one to two cups a day. During the first few days, the caffeine withdrawal symptoms might give you a headache. Counteract this with two litres of liquid (water or herbal tea), as well as one or two 400-milligram magnesium tablets per day. If you really don't want to give up on coffee, then at least try not to drink any in the afternoon. This will help you to feel calmer in the evening and to fall asleep more easily. It may be tough, but make a point of really savouring the one or two cups you drink in the morning. Later in the day, switch to beverages such as herbal tea or sparkling water.

During perimenopause, and especially if you are suffering from CAI, it is worth giving up coffee for a while. Only then can you find out what effect coffee has on you. If you notice that without coffee you feel more stable, experience fewer hot flushes, suffer less from oestrogen dominance, sleep better, and are less restless and anxious, then decide if and why you need coffee (to wake up, for stimulation, for pleasure, for social reasons). Based on this knowledge, decide on a reduced daily amount. You will soon realise that you feel fine with it.

A daily schedule for adrenal exhaustion

- Vitamin C 1,000 milligrams per day
- Vitamin B complex once a day
- Magnesium citrate, two times 300 milligrams per day (reduce to one time 300 milligrams if your stool grows soft, as magnesium has a laxative effect)
- Omega 3 fatty acids two times 1,000 milligrams per day
- Asian ginseng
- Ashwagandha 200 milligrams per day
- Liquorice root extract 200 milligrams per day

If cortisol is administered directly (which is necessary in individual cases, for example, in cases of burnout syndrome, when the adrenal cortex is completely 'worn out'), the symptoms disappear quickly. Only natural hydrocortisone should be used in these cases. For asthma, rheumatism, or other diseases where the aim is to intentionally suppress an overshooting immune system, strongly effective corticosteroids are often used — but not in the case of adrenal insufficiency.

DHEA progesterone: In the case of adrenal exhaustion, DHEA is available as a drug for men. Women are better off taking progesterone; this increases the DHEA level indirectly.

Balance: Work on creating physical and mental balance, even on a biochemical level. Ideally, in every single cell of the body, the processes of building and breaking down are balanced. This requires alternation of action and rest, of enjoyable meals and breaks from eating, as well as a healthy sleeping-and-waking rhythm. If we were to turn night into day all the time, our bodies would not last long. Because sleep is the best cure, not only for stress, we want to give our sleep cycles a special section.

CHRONOBIOLOGY — PRESCRIPTION SLEEPING

All living things on our planet, even protozoa and plants, have an internal clock. It is dependent on the day–night rhythm, on light and darkness, on the seasons, and also the lunar cycle. All bodily functions are permanently adapted to this inner clock, known as the circadian rhythm. You could also say that when in balance, our insides work like a Swiss watch. It is not only the sleep rhythm that is adapted to day-and-night phases, but also the production of hormones, metabolic processes, temperature regulation, and even our emotions. This archaic, natural mechanism is anchored in our genes.

Jeffrey C. Hall, Michael Rosbash, and Michael W. Young were awarded the Nobel Prize for Medicine in 2017 for their study of the internal clock. In that study, they point out that before electricity was invented, people went to bed at the same time as their chickens and got up with them too. The fields were cultivated according to the seasons. Meals were made up of whatever had just been harvested, slaughtered, or hunted, or whatever else nature provided. Summer fruits were preserved for the winter, and potatoes and apples were stored in a dark place. The holes in trousers were mended by candlelight in the evening, while telling each other the stories of the day. That old lifestyle may have been less romantic than we sometimes imagine it, but what is certain is that by 8.00 pm or 9.00 pm, everyone was tucked up in bed.

Since the invention of electricity, nothing has been the same. The light bulb and the steam engine have catapulted our organism out of its evolutionary cycle. Since then, human beings have turned night into day. Night shifts were introduced, and people work around the clock all over the world. Aeroplanes can cross time zones. In a few years, anyone who can afford to will be able to fly to Mars. The fact that our body shouts out: 'Whew! Stop! Are you crazy?' is not surprising, for although it is excellent at adapting, there are limits.

This is why in shift work and prolonged lack of sleep there is an increased risk not only of infection, but also of some types of cancer.

Repair processes that take place mainly during rest are suppressed. As a result, genetic changes (mutations) cannot be sufficiently remedied. This is why, apart from presenting an increased cancer risk, sleep deprivation can also cause headaches, high blood pressure, cardiovascular diseases, and a weakened immune system.

According to a report carried out by the German Health Employees' Health Insurance (DAK) in 2017, 34 million people in Germany suffer from sleep disorders; 35 per cent of the working population said that they struggle to fall asleep or to sleep through the night three to four times a week. One in ten menopausal women complains of sleep problems.

This is why stress needs to be properly addressed, along with the sleep hormone melatonin.

Melatonin

Melatonin comes from the pineal gland, a small gland in the diencephalon, as well as being distributed in the retina of the eyes and in the intestine. It takes over the night shift in our bodies and rocks us to sleep, so to speak. Darkness is the signal for the distribution. When it gets light outside again, the production of melatonin, which is 12 times as high during the night compared to the day, is suppressed. This is why we wake up.

Hence, we struggle to fall asleep when we stare into the bright screen of our tablet to check the latest news or watch television before going to bed. The brightness of the light source throws our pineal gland off balance; it thinks it is time to get up, and reduces the melatonin. The blue wavelengths are particularly problematic as they perk us up just like caffeine. You don't notice them because the screen on your tablet looks whitish. Two hours of work at a computer screen reduces melatonin production by a fifth. No wonder you can't fall asleep! Modern tablets and mobile phones have a blue light filter, which allows you to switch off this particular type of light.

Melatonin receptors are found in the heart, kidneys, immune cells, the spleen, the retina, the blood vessels of the brain, and the liver (in which the sleep hormone is also broken down). Melatonin also lowers our body temperature. Studies have shown that melatonin also influences other hormones, has an anti-inflammatory effect, and stimulates cell regeneration. The breakdown in the liver leads to intermediate products that protect against free radicals.

From around the age of 40, we produce only 60 per cent of the melatonin that an adolescent produces. This natural deficiency of the sleep hormone then causes nocturnal disturbance. The circadian rhythm is also significantly influenced by alcohol, coffee, stress, hormonal changes, and strong temperature fluctuations. In addition, each person has their own biorhythm — some hop out of bed easily in the mornings, while others are night owls.

Owl or lark?

Studies have shown that the biorhythm of most people can be split into two categories: early risers, known as larks, and those who are not at their best until early afternoon or evening, known as owls. Teenagers going through puberty tend to be late risers, so they are owls. Any parent who has spent years repeatedly waking up their sleepy teens for school in the mornings will not need a scientific study to tell them this.

Over the course of life, the biorhythm changes. This will be familiar to all parents when you think back to when your children were little. You were probably keen for a few hours more sleep when your two-year-old would come and tug at your arm at 6.00 am and wouldn't rest until you read them their favourite book again.

Our chronobiology is particularly susceptible to disruptive factors during phases of hormonal change. Lack of sleep influences our concentration, feelings of satiety, metabolic processes, performance, the energy which we (no longer) have available, and not least, our nerves. Sleep becomes ever more important for the body — you can recognise this by the fact that you might be able to deal with one all-nighter, but definitely not two.

SKB: 'It takes me longer to recover from a seminar or three or four exhausting workdays in a row. If I get up at seven, spend the whole day non-stop in meetings or surrounded by people and then have a professional event or a dinner in the evenings, then I fall into bed bone-weary at midnight. Especially when I am travelling, for days afterwards I feel the lack of sleep and the exhaustion in my bones, if not in every single cell. Meanwhile, after a seminar, I consciously cancel everything from my diary that starts before 10.00 am, so that I can try to catch up on some sleep. Or I'll go for a walk in the woods or around the lake in the mornings to recharge my batteries.'

During the time of hormonal change, it is important to recognise your own altered needs and not carry on with business as usual. What has worked for many years — little sleep or working through an overly full appointment calendar — may work for a little while, but eventually it comes back to bite you at the expense of your health. It is not worth it. If you familiarise yourself with your altered biorhythm, you will get through the day with less stress, feeling more harmonious, balanced, and relaxed. Then you can see your own needs in a totally different light. No longer 'higher, further, faster' at the expense of your health and definitely not with the feeling of failing or being undisciplined or lazy. Our body signals that it has had enough, that it needs more sleep, and that it needs to retreat from the hustle and bustle for a moment during the day to recharge. It doesn't want to annoy us — on the contrary, it wants to protect us! So, should we not give it the opportunity to work for us instead of demanding more and more from it? Observe your own rhythm for a week and then to the fullest extent possible for you, decide to live it, bit by bit. This is not going to work from one day to the next. Sleeping until 10.00 am, taking a walk at lunchtime or lying down in a meadow and watching the clouds drift by, taking an hour for afternoon tea and then going to bed with a good book at 9.00 pm is an unrealistic dream for many. But it may be possible to integrate into our everyday life one or two more relaxing habits, which then also improve our sleep. And please do this without a guilty conscience! Read about how to do this in Chapter 5.

Sleeping pills

Under no circumstances should you take sleeping pills without discussing it with your doctor. Talk to them about your specific sleep issues: do you find it difficult to fall asleep, do you lie awake worrying, do you wake up several times during the night and feel wrecked the next morning?

SLEEP STRATEGIES

- Become the expert on your inner clock!
- Your day dictates how you sleep. If you are on the go all day, then you will struggle to fall asleep.
- Spend as much time as possible outdoors during the day, even on days when the sky is overcast. This not only promotes vitamin D production, but also suppresses melatonin and makes you more alert.
- Almost all cultures swear by going to sleep before midnight.
- The bedroom should be cool, dark, and quiet.
- Ban all electronic devices from the bedroom. Mobile phones must at least be in flight mode or, better still, turned off.
- Do not use digital devices before falling asleep, or if absolutely necessary, activate the blue-light filter. The pineal gland will not react as strongly to this warmer light.
- Do not watch horror movies or anything so tense that it will set your body into alarm mode before going to bed.
- Do not check your emails before going to bed. This means you are less likely to lie awake brooding.
- The cortisol level is at its highest approximately one to two

hours after waking up and allows us to launch ourselves dynamically into the day. As cortisol is also released during intense sporting activity, and the stimulating effect lasts for several hours, it is a good idea not to do any sport or vigorous exercise after 7.00 pm. After this hour, if you feel like doing some exercise, consider doing a gentle yoga practice, which calms the system.

- Consuming a rich, heavy, or very late meal in the evening also affects the quality of our sleep. You should be especially careful to avoid fat, highly processed sugar, and carbohydrates — these lead to increased insulin release with subsequent hypoglycaemia, which means you will probably wake up during the night with your stomach growling.

- The stimulant caffeine lowers melatonin levels and therefore logically makes falling asleep more difficult. So, do without the espresso in the evening and switch to decaf alternatives such as herbal tea.

- Sometimes a hot water bottle, a small wheat bag, or wearing woolly socks in bed can help prevent you from waking up during the night — even if it is not very sexy. Or if you have a partner, you can of course also cuddle up to them.

- A recipe that our grandmothers used was warm milk with honey before bedtime. There is something to be said for this, as milk contains melatonin and tryptophan, both in very low quantities, but many generations have benefited from it. Caffeine-free chai tea (without black tea in it), or 'golden milk' (milk simmered with turmeric) also works.

There are many medical and psychological reasons why you might struggle to get much rest at night. Sleep disturbances can, for example, be an early sign of depression. In some cases, it might be possible to find out the cause by spending some time in a sleep lab.

Melatonin is freely available to buy in many countries around the world, for example, in the US, but it requires a prescription in Germany and is only permitted for primary sleep disorders (a sleep disorder that is not associated with another disease). We advise against purchasing melatonin online and using it as a treatment method without discussing this with your doctor first. The long-term effects have not been fully tested yet.

Benzodiazepines sedate, but they have a high potential for dependency. They may only be used for short periods of time for acute sleep disorders and should only be given on medical advice. They are effectively very low-dose antidepressants that promote sleep.

Bioidentical progesterone calms. This is why, in HRT, it makes sense to take progesterone in the evenings.

Many herbs have a calming or sleep-inducing effect. These include valerian, hops, lavender, passionflower, and yellow sweet clover. The herbs are available in the form of tea, in pillows, oils, tinctures, and tablets. Ask your pharmacist which herb in which preparation might help best with your sleeping disorder.

LIVER DETOXIFICATION

The adrenal gland is not the only organ that is affected by permanent stress; the liver also struggles. And we particularly need its support during this time of hormonal adjustment.

The liver is the body's detoxification centre, and this function means it has to sort and clear through unimaginable amounts of material. There is hardly a substance or a medicine that is not tested or disassembled here. Pathogens and toxins are rendered harmless in the liver, and, above all, most of our hormones, such as oestrogen, progesterone, and thyroid hormones, are broken down here.

In order to cope with this, the liver works around the clock — and woe betide us if it doesn't. Lack of exercise and, with it, poor circulation, but also a diet too rich in fat or sugar as well as regular alcohol consumption are just some of the reasons why liver diseases such as fatty liver, liver fibrosis, and liver cirrhosis are on the rise. But as the liver does not complain when it is not feeling well, these diseases are often only recognised very late.

We advise you to look after your liver and regularly give it a detox. This also indirectly affects all the hormone glands such as the adrenal and thyroid glands. If you take regular detox days where you abstain from alcohol, sugar, and fat, then your liver will be in seventh heaven. On those days drink at least two litres of green, unsweetened tea. Eat a lot of natural bitter substances, such as artichoke, milk thistle, and dandelion leaves. That also makes for a happy liver.

LIVER WRAP TREATMENT

Make a hot liver wrap before bedtime. This stimulates the blood circulation and therefore detoxification. It's best to do this treatment for seven consecutive nights. Place a hot, damp cloth under your right ribcage, and put a hot water bottle over it. Wrap this around you with a towel and let it sit for half an hour. A brew of yarrow (a medicinal plant that stimulates the digestive organs) is recommended for soaking the cloth.

During this time, make yourself comfortable on the sofa or in bed with a good book, watching your favourite TV show or just relaxing. This is pure heaven.

4

External Hormone Manipulation

Endocrine disrupters

In the previous chapters we have shown how hormones control our body and how we can use them to support our health. Now let's look at the saboteurs who are secretly destroying our hormone system 'from the outside'. Chemicals and artificial compounds gain access to our bodies through food packaging, clothing, cosmetics, and the air we breathe. These so-called endocrine disruptors disrupt our fragile natural hormone cycle. In addition, these substances have the potential to change not only our genetic makeup during our lifetime, but also that of our children and grandchildren. Meanwhile the data shows that 90 per cent of the population in the western industrialised countries are polluted with hormone-active substances.

In 2012, the World Health Organization (WHO) categorised endocrine disruptors as a global threat. Its definition reads: 'Endocrine disruptors are externally delivered substances or mixtures that interfere with the functioning of the hormone system and therefore cause harmful effects on health in an intact organism, in their offspring or in (partial) populations.'

For a long time now, scientists and doctors have been observing a dramatic increase in the number of diseases associated with a hormone system that is out of sync. Like the WHO, the German Society of Endocrinology (DGE) has been pointing out for years that hormone-active chemicals affect our health by damaging the hormone system and the metabolism. The society says that endocrine disruptors can cause hormone-triggered diseases like breast cancer and prostate cancer. They can compromise the nervous system of children, and some believe that they can also contribute to the development of attention deficit hyperactivity disorder (ADHD). Malformations of the genitalia as well as reduced sperm production were also cited by the DGE. It is also suspected that the sharp global increase in thyroid and metabolic diseases, like diabetes mellitus and excess weight, are not solely due to a genetic predisposition or an unhealthy lifestyle, but that endocrine disruptors also play a causal role. The DGE therefore advises that these substances should be used with extreme caution.

BUT HOW DO THESE ARTIFICIAL HORMONE MODULATORS WORK?

DGE media spokesman Professor Helmut Schatz explains that endocrine disruptors upset the balance of the hormone system, the immune system, the metabolism, fat storage, and bone development. Acting like endogenous hormones, endocrine disruptors have a big influence on the endocrine system as exogenous chemicals and can cause lasting disruption. They can dysregulate our system in much the same way that synthetic hormones can. Endocrine disrupters or their chemical elements bind themselves to the receptors of the endogenous hormones. There, they either trigger the same reaction as the 'right' hormone, which in fact is not wanted at that time, or they block the receptor and prevent the endogenous hormones from docking on. In addition, they can disrupt the production, transport, and breakdown of endogenous hormones and change their concentration. Endocrine disrupters can lead to oestrogen dominance along with its associated symptoms and diseases, described in Chapter 3.

> SEB: 'For certain symptoms and disorders I ask my patients to bring all the cosmetic products from their bathroom and/ or to write down all the substances that they are in contact with in the home. You wouldn't believe the endless lists and the amount of pollutants that are contained on these products.'

Endocrine disrupters are also known as *environmental hormones*. This term is doubly unfortunate, because the endocrine disrupters are by no means the same as endogenous hormones, and the word 'environment' is also out of place here. To some, the word 'environment' makes them think of 'nature', but there's nothing 'natural' about these products. The chemicals simply mimic the hormones. Their effects on the body are anything but wholesome. In 2013, leading health scientists appealed to the European Union in the form of the Berlaymont Declaration, asking for a new way of dealing with endocrine disrupters. In their estimation, even very small doses have a damaging effect, especially when they build up in the body. So stricter regulations are essential. Further studies are already in progress in order to precisely assess the risks.

An example of endocrine disrupters is bisphenol A (BPA), which is contained in plastic and used as food packaging. This chemical is the most widely produced in the world and we will look at it in more detail later. Aluminium is another of at least 800 chemical substances in our everyday life that affects hormone cycles. Aluminium is suspected of increasing the risk of breast cancer and Alzheimer's disease; even though there is no statistically significant evidence, manufacturers of common brands have stopped using aluminium in their cosmetic products. Dichlorodiphenyltrichloroethane (DDT), now a banned pesticide, increases soil erosion and will be washed out of the soil for many years to come. Glyphosate is currently the most controversial pesticide; it has caused a great deal of trouble for global corporations. Phthalates are plasticisers that provide elasticity and bendability to plastics and are contained in floor coverings, food packaging, paints, imitation leather, and children's toys. The Federal Ministry for Environment and Nature in Germany has said that plasticisers have a hormone-like effect and can influence the human hormonal system. They are particularly dangerous in that they are not firmly bound in the plastic. When heated, they evaporate, and can be inhaled or absorbed through food. Phthalates are classified as toxic to the liver and are thought to trigger obesity and diabetes. A 2015 study carried out on mice by researchers at the University of Leipzig showed that the mice that drank water containing plasticisers for ten weeks got fat despite being given normal food. This proves that plasticisers can disrupt sugar metabolism. The term 'obesogens' — obesity-causing substances in plastic and other products — is commonly used in relation to plasticisers today, analogous to the term 'teratogens' for carcinogens, substances that cause cancer. Cadmium can be found in some toys. Triclosans are found in antibacterial products and toothpastes, and parabens in cosmetic products.

> SEB: 'When we are treating patients, we must consider the hormonal shifts caused by the daily use of plastics. What good is a change of diet or a diet for weight reduction if the BPA from the food packaging of the yoghurt affects the fat metabolism? I wonder if in future we might find a question on medical history questionnaires asking about patients' consumer behaviour. This is really interesting. Research in the field must and will continue to be a priority for us in the coming years. It's unlikely to give the all-clear. My advice is: don't rely on legislation. Try to avoid plastic and microplastic as much as possible. This is in the interests of your own health and it also protects the environment.'

BPA is used as a plasticiser and gelling agent in many everyday items such as plastic-coated cans, beer and soft-drink cans, plastic drink bottles, Tetra Pak, packaging for shrink-wrapped vegetables, plastic-coated shopping receipts, plastic spectacles, and much, much more. Through heat, BPA gets into food — for example, by heating plastic containers in the microwave or when a plastic bottle stands in the sun for too long. BPA contains fat-soluble properties and is therefore quickly absorbed into the body and stored in the fatty tissue. An American study has shown that just a few days after consumption of food that was packaged in coated plastics, a BPA value 20 times the normal level showed up in urine tests. What is so worrying about this is the fact that BPA has oestrogen-like effects that can lead to premature puberty and behavioural issues in children. Due to significantly increased BPA blood levels found in women with polycystic ovarian syndrome, some people believe there is an association between this hormone disorder and endocrine disrupters.

Japan has had BPA-free canned foods on the market for 20 years. France has had a national ban on BPA in all materials that come into contact with food since 2015. Germany is lagging behind, even though the Federal Environment Agency welcomes the EU's decision to recognise BPA as being of particular concern because of its hormonal effects on animals and the environment. Thermal paper, like that used in sales receipts, has been prohibited throughout the EU since 2020. From 2021, products such as plastic plates and cutlery, straws, and cotton swabs made of plastic etc. for which there are safe alternatives, will disappear from the EU market.

Plastic is a chemical cocktail that is largely made from endocrine disrupters. Microplastics are particularly dangerous.

MICROPLASTICS

Microplastics are plastic particles that are smaller than five millimetres across. Microplastic is contained in synthetic textiles, in the particles that wear away from car tyres, in shower gel, shampoo, toothpaste, exfoliants, children's toys, and thousands of other everyday objects, and is released by the decomposition of packaging. Microplastic is indestructible and has been found in the earth's most remote areas, washed up via wastewater and sea currents. Scientists were even able to find microplastic in form of polypropylene (PP) and polyethylene terephthalate (PET) at the North and South Poles.

Primary microplastics are produced in the form of microspheres, which are added to cosmetics and cleaning products as well as fleece and other plastics for clothing. Over 300,000 tons of microplastic, which survive any sewage plant treatment, are released across Germany annually. The stuff gets into fields, rivers, and seas via sewage sludge. Eventually it can be swallowed by fish that might end up on our dinner plate. In 2019, researchers published the results of an Austrian pilot study. Within the framework of this study, microplastic was found, for the first time, in human intestines. The study participants (aged 35 to 65) came from different continents. During the study, all food stuffs, including fish and seafood, were packaged in plastic, and the drinks in PET bottles. For one week, the test subjects wrote down everything they ate and drank, and then gave a stool sample. The result: ten grams of stool contained an average of 20 particles of microplastic!

Unfortunately, microplastic particles draw toxins from the environment like a magnet attracts paperclips, and, in just the same way, the pollutants stick to them. Even chemicals that have been banned for a long time, such as DDT, are still found in high concentrations in the food chain.

Secondary microplastics are the product of decay and weathering of large plastic parts, such as bottles, bags, and other plastic waste that floats around the ocean and gets into the environment. Incidentally, the abrasion caused by car tyres is responsible for the largest share of microplastics in the air. Clothes are another environmental and health polluter. Over 70 per cent of all textiles contain synthetic fibres such as elastane, polyethylene, and polyester — found in the lining of winter jackets, in multifunctional clothing, sweat-repellent sportswear, and weatherproof jackets, among other things. Microplastic particles are released with each wash and make their way into the oceans and the bellies of fish through washing machine wastewater, via the route we mentioned earlier. Students from the Karlsruhe Institute of Technology in Germany developed a microplastic filter and presented it to the public in 2019. It is hoped that in future these young researchers might be able to work with an industrial partner so that their invention can become a standard part of all washing machines.

Plastic packaging poses a particular problem. Products are added to the plastic to make it both flexible and strong, or to give it a special colour. Some plastic bottles contain over 1,500 ingredients. Only the plastic industry knows the exact composition of most plastic packaging, and they don't talk about it. As diseases of western civilisation such as hormonal imbalances, allergies, cardiovascular diseases, asthma, and diabetes are increasing at the same furious rate as plastic production and waste, there is a growing suspicion that there might be a connection. Researchers now believe that the particles which come from the food packaging and pass to the food products are potentially — if not definitely — damaging to our health.

One potential danger, as already mentioned, is that plastics emit substances. We inhale or ingest these emissions that mix with the dust in our houses.

SEB: 'We recently disposed of all products that contain plastic in our household. This quickly made a surprisingly huge pile of pots, jars, packaging, and containers on the living room floor. Initially, when we went shopping, we only looked out for products that were free of microplastic. Then we realised that there was no point buying high-quality cosmetics in polluting plastic packaging. Firstly, they add to the huge mountains of rubbish, and secondly, they might emit endocrine disruptors and other chemical substances. We have changed the way we shop, and we have had to say goodbye to many products, some of which we miss a great deal, others less so. And to be honest, many of the things that are considered indispensable, we didn't miss at all. It also resulted in some funny situations. The first attempts at replacing our shampoo with a bar of soap led to matted hair. No one in the family dared to leave the house afterwards. Meanwhile, there are great alternatives in the shops such as solid shampoo and conditioner bars. They work. Over time, everyone in the family was able to find healthy and sustainable alternatives. It also helps to ask the sales assistants which products are free of microplastics and pollutants. The more customers that ask for these products, the more likely it is that the products will be changed for the better.'

REDUCE, RE-USE, RECYCLE

As consumers we have varying amounts of choice about what we spend our money on and the risks we want to expose ourselves to, depending on how privileged we are. You do not have to turn your entire life upside down, but with a few small changes you can do a lot for your own health and to protect the environment. More and more of us are trying to reduce our consumption, purchase products in recyclable packaging, and re-use as much as we can, including our shopping bags.

- Avoid plastic wherever possible and avoid single-use items.
- Pay attention to the ingredients. The products should be: phthalate-free, BPA-free, paraben-free. With the app 'Scan4Chem' you can find out from the manufacturer which endocrine disrupters are included in the product.
- Take your fabric bags with you to the shops (the many paper

bags that end up in the recycling bin at home don't really help the environment, either).

- Use BPA-free containers for leftover food, and avoid using cling film or aluminium foil.
- Buy unpacked vegetables instead of, for example, shrink-wrapped cucumbers or plastic punnets of tomatoes. In many supermarkets now, you can buy unpackaged produce, and of course you can do the same if you shop at markets.
- Do not heat any food that has previously been wrapped in plastic.
- Avoid drinks in plastic bottles and cans.
- Do not buy tins that are lined with plastic.
- Avoid cosmetic products, perfumes, room sprays, and air fresheners that contain synthetic fragrances. Use essential oils instead.
- Use a protective net bag when washing your clothes in the washing machine.
- Try to buy clothes made of natural fibres rather than synthetic fibres.
- Use water filters to treat your drinking water.

Studies in recent years have clearly shown that endocrine disrupters are passed on via the placenta into the bloodstream of the foetus, as well as through breast milk. These children may be at increased risk of various diseases later on in life. It's important that anyone who wants to have children is aware of this, so that they can make an informed decision. Even if this no longer affects you, it could affect your friends, daughters, and granddaughters of childbearing age. As we mentioned at the beginning, endocrine disrupters and other dangerous chemicals find their way into our genes. Let's take a closer look at this.

Epigenetics —
from the environment to the genes

For a long time, it was believed that everything was determined for us by the time we were in the womb: eye colour, character, predisposition to certain diseases, and so on. 'It's in their genes, there is nothing you can do,' was the credo. But is it true that humans are nothing but the sum of their genes? Far from it!

Today we know that we are not just at the mercy of our genetic destiny. On the contrary: environmental factors, nutrition, our life experiences, and many other influences can switch certain genes in the cell nucleus on or off at any time. The science that studies and proves this phenomenon is called epigenetics (composed of the word *epigenesis* — the development of a living being — and *genetics*).

Epigenetics studies the influence of the environment on genes and has led to a radical rethink. In terms of health, only 20 per cent of the influence of our genes is fixed. The remaining 80 per cent is influenced by our living conditions, eating habits, environment, and so on. Even minor lifestyle changes can interfere with our genetic material. According to the latest research, this also affects changes in our personality traits. So, an angry or grumpy person cannot blame their genes for the rest of their life.

By understanding epigenetics, researchers hope to find answers to the big questions of medicine: how are behaviour and experiences stored in our cells, and why, out of two random people who have a cancer gene, for example, does only one get ill and the other doesn't? Epigenetics investigates the causes of the diseases. This is why it is considered one of the most promising branches of medical research.

But epigenetics also plays an important role in the treatment of diseases. Why is a drug extremely effective in one patient, and less effective or associated with severe side effects in another? These are called intra-individual differences. Or: what is the cause of a chronic disease? Which structural options are there, what support is needed, where can individualised therapies be applied and when will they help?

THE BLUEPRINT OF OUR LIFE

Every human being has about 25,000 to 50,000 genes, which together are described as the human genome. This was completely decrypted in the Human Genome Project from 1990 to 2003. There are 46 chromosomes in each human somatic cell nucleus — apart from in the red blood cells. These chromosomes consist of a chemical structure that contains bases, sugars, and phosphate: the DNA — deoxyribonucleic acid. It contains the entire genetic information to be stored in individual sections, the genes. The DNA of all people on the earth — whether fat, thin, tall, small, blond or red-haired, blue-eyed or green-eyed — is 99 per cent identical! That uniqueness that we consider so important is, genetically speaking, extremely minimal.

DNA lies spirally in the cell nucleus as a double strand; stretched out it is about two metres long and contains the largest alphabet in the world: 6.54 billion genetic letters. It is our hardware, so to speak, and has a storage capacity that is bigger than any computer chip. For those who like an analogy: on the pinhead-sized DNA, the content of all books ever written would only take up a fraction of the memory space. However, only a tiny fraction of it is used, or perhaps we don't yet have the technology to know what the rest is actually good for.

DNA is also known as genetic code or fingerprinting. Words (sequences) are formed from the individual genetic letters, which code the protein structures (amino acids). These swarm out into the body and bring about everything that makes a human being and everything that is necessary to survive. This includes cell regeneration, cell breakdown, messenger substances, hormones, organ function, and so on. In other words: inside each cell nucleus is your own personal instruction manual. Here you will find replenishment

OUR HORMONES, OUR HEALTH

for hair that has fallen out, for grazed skin on your knee, for plucked eyebrows, for hormones and much, much more.

In order to understand epigenetics, it is important to know that genes can be switched on and off. Let's stick with the image of the gigantic library: epigenetics is like a bookmark that you put in a book to find the page or gene on the DNA. This labelling is used to switch genes on or off and to start or end the production of protein structures. This process is called methylation. Small molecules, methyl groups, signal, 'That's enough now.' They block a specific section of the gene on the DNA strand and prevent any action there. This section cannot be read, and the information therefore not translated into a protein. This gene segment, or the gene itself, is therefore virtually switched off. Conversely, sections can be labelled where genes are switched on.

The methyl groups are influenced by environmental factors. These markers can permanently anchor themselves in the genome and can accordingly be passed on. This makes epigenetics something like the turbo engine of evolution, because in just one generation a large part of the genetic heritage can change in this way.

Proof of the heritability of acquired traits was provided by the Swiss molecular biologist Renato Paro in 2004. He and his team treated fruit flies with external heat. As a result, the fruit flies grew red eyes instead of white ones, and their offspring also had red eyes, despite the fact that they were not exposed to the heat.

WE CAN ACTIVELY MODIFY OUR GENES

Armed with information, we have a great amount of power to influence our genes. They don't just control us; we can control them too. Health is therefore less of a fixed destiny than previously thought.

We can use epigenetics to make a profound difference to our bodies. We can make meaningful changes to stay healthy and vital for as long as possible. An example we saw at the beginning of this chapter is to avoid endocrine disrupters (see page 205).

We do not want to make people who aren't able to make lots of changes in their lives feel guilty or fearful. The influences that determine our health are complex. In Chapter 3, we showed just how complex the hormone cycles are. Knowing about epigenetics, though, can motivate us to make a difference to our health. Especially in perimenopause, understanding epigenetics can help us move towards a deeper understanding of our own bodies.

As far as foods go, the superstars of epigenetics are avocados, broccoli, pomegranates, salad, whole grains, leafy green vegetables, beans, liver, and fatty fish. They contain important vitamins, including the entire vitamin B group. Vitamin D, which is formed in the skin when we spend time outdoors, is an epigenetic booster too. Healthy nutrition and a healthy lifestyle therefore not only protect our own health, but could also influence the health of our children, grandchildren, and great-grandchildren.

The groundbreaking new scientific findings from this branch of research impressively demonstrate how our actions and decisions affect the blueprint of our lives. According to a Finnish study among a group of men, daily 20-minute sauna sessions over a four-week period led to a 50-per-cent drop in the risk of developing cardio-vascular disease. The warmth switched off a particular gene. The influence of social relationships is also significant to the epigenome, in a lasting way. Newborn babies who don't have enough human contact — whether from their parents or another constant caregiver — have greater problems forming attachments in adulthood and are more likely to develop biologically detectable disorders within their stress-hormone system. It is safe to assume that almost any disease has an epigenetic component.

Every seven years almost all cells in the body renew themselves. This means we consist of new building blocks every seven years and

are therefore our own master builders. We should use this opportunity and provide our bodies with outstanding building material.
This includes adequate sleep, stress reduction, self-care practices,
outdoor exercise, healthy food (locally produced, seasonal, and
unpackaged wherever possible), and the avoidance of endocrine
disruptors and microplastics.

> SEB: 'Stress management and sufficient sleep especially help
> to protect our genes. I have seen many times that people are
> much kinder to themselves when they realise how much
> better it is for their health.'

This is exactly what the next chapter is about — good self-care.

5

Self-care

You will inevitably take on many roles throughout your life. As a daughter, sibling, partner, lover, professional, homemaker, or parent, you will give some Oscar-worthy performances. Sometimes your life may feel like a soap opera, sometimes a comedy, a tragedy, a romcom, or even a thriller. And you'll probably be playing many of these roles simultaneously.

Every task in life has its moment. Especially during the time when hormones are changing, almost all women rethink their own role or the roles they have played for so long. In the best-case scenario, you were convincing, joyful, and fulfilled in your role, but perhaps occasionally with the feeling that your life was not under your control and you were acting out of a sense of duty. Many women have been culturally conditioned to be extremely good at switching from one role to another and putting everyone else's needs above their own.

Interestingly, the beginning of the hormone roller-coaster often coincides with the phase in life when some women start to feel they have had enough of their role as caregivers within the family, in their community, or in the office. In a restaurant, we recently overheard a woman in her mid-forties at the next table say: 'I'm shutting up shop at home; I am so fed up of caring for everyone and being responsible for everything.'

If you are one of those people who suddenly realises that they are no longer the first to put up their hand to volunteer for the parent-teacher association or any extra work going in the office, this may have something to do with your evolutionary 'provider hormones' decreasing. Don't feel guilty about this. This might be nature's way of letting you know that you need to conserve your energy instead of giving it all away.

In this chapter we will being giving you a lot of suggestions on how to set boundaries, how to say *no*, and how to put a stop to things that drain your energy.

To identify who and what is draining your energy, we will keep asking you questions for self-reflection like: *what do you need in order to feel well? How would you like to feel (again)? Who do you want to be and, more importantly, who do you no longer want to be? What are your plans for the future? What things are on your wish list? Which of your many roles no longer suits you?*

Maybe you've been responsible for your family and friends for many years. Now it is time to take responsibility for yourself. This process supports the holistic approach to preventing illness. If we are always there for others, but never for ourselves, then this negatively influences our own health.

Recently, a friend said to me: 'Life is not a dress rehearsal, it's the premiere.' In this sense, menopause is the next exciting act for the development of your own personality. The stage is set for the wonderful opportunity to take your own needs seriously and to think about what you want.

Imagine falling in love at first sight. You enter into the relationship with a huge leap of faith, seeing everything in a rosy, romantic hue. Isn't it a wonderful feeling? And now imagine that you are seeing yourself with the same kindness and generosity of spirit. We don't mean this in the sense of becoming narcissistic, but just the sense of getting rid of those unconscious self-destructive beliefs that prevent many of us from becoming the person that they are, deep within themselves.

Often this approach can be blocked by negative experiences or beliefs like 'I should be perfect, I'm not good enough or not beautiful enough.' But in mid-life in particular, a lot of women are able to lift this black curtain in order to discover the real 'me' backstage. This is not only extremely good for our mental health but also presents surprising insights. You discover a new way of being, which brings fresh energy to the old 'me'. And with that, you can step curiously and joyfully into the coming years. By looking at the problems in your life closely, you can take full responsibility for your own part in them and move towards some healthy, self-nurturing change. This can include addressing anger, pain, or loss, as well as grief about the fact that we are leaving certain parts of our life behind. The storms and crises of the midlife phase should not be underestimated, but they provide a huge opportunity to finally tackle the things close to our hearts.

This also undoubtedly includes a great deal of self-care, including loving relationships, which from a medical perspective — alongside stress reduction and a healthy diet — also strengthen the endocrine system. Some parts of our life need to be addressed now, especially those that are no longer helpful for us. They may require us to change course, or at least give them some attention. However, the path you will take is always as individual and adaptable as life itself. What works for one person might not be an option for another — and vice versa.

We hope that by the end of this chapter, and by the end of the book, you have a clearer understanding of yourself and your wishes, and that you will be kinder, more forgiving, and more generous to yourself in the future. Good health, contentment, and a new lightness of spirit are the reward for exploring what you need for your own body and mind. Out of the hormonal chaos and into life!

To this end, we would like to start with some questions for you. Sit and relax in your favourite place, perhaps with a cup of tea or coffee and some good music, while you answer them. We want you to consciously focus on the long positive list (and not on the negative list). It might be necessary to take a new perspective here in order to look at yourself in the same way you would look at someone you are in love with. If this is too tricky for you, try viewing yourself the way that you'd view a dear friend, or someone in your life who you care deeply about.

Write the answers down in a nice notebook.

QUESTIONNAIRE

1. What do you like about yourself? (Please write everything down!)
    a. Character (e.g. I am reliable)
    b. External (e.g. my eyes)
2. What do you value in your life? (Please write everything down!)
3. What are you really proud of?
4. Are you in a relationship?
    a. If you are, do you feel your partner treats you with respect? Are you cherished and loved? Are you happy in your relationship?
    b. Have you given up on your relationship because it's just not the same as it used to be?
    c. Do you still have hopes and dreams that your relationship might be revitalised, happier and more erotic again? For b) and c), write down five things that you want in the relationship (e.g. more or less sex, more tenderness, respect, attention, interest) and plan on talking to your partner about it. Have an open discussion about your own needs — this is doctor's orders!

5. Is your sex life — with your partner and/or yourself — fulfilling?

6. If you are employed, do you like going to work? Do you enjoy your job?

7. Have you found your life's work? What is it? And if not, what could it be?

8. Do you consider your life meaningful? What could give it more purpose?

9. Are you creative? Do you want to be? If not, what is stopping you?

10. If you could have one wish, what would it be?

11. Would you like to break out of some aspect of your life? If yes, from where? What is stopping you?

12. Do you know what would make you happy? If you are not happy and you know what would make you happy, what's standing in the way?

13. Do you feel enough love, self-love, friendship, excitement, hope, and longing?

14. Are there still things you dream of doing? (Please write them down, regardless of how realistic they are at this point.)

15. Are you good to yourself? Can you protect yourself against overload, set limits, articulate your needs, and assert yourself?

16. Do you regularly ask yourself what it is that you want?

17. Can you accept help? Is there an area in your life for which you absolutely need help (e.g. with the care of a relative, in your household, during arguments with your teenage children)?

18. Do you get enough peace and quiet? Do you take regular short or long breaks?

19. Do you live in peace with those around you (work, family, friends, neighbours)? If not, would you consider seeking the help of a professional (mediator, counsellor, psychologist)?

20. Is your financial situation secure? If not, are there any

OUR HORMONES, OUR HEALTH

changes you could make to improve the situation (e.g. asking for a pay rise, working extra hours, cancelling redundant insurance or subscriptions, selling things that have been gathering dust in your loft, downsizing, taking public transport instead of driving a car), and where could you save money (buying second-hand, changing your food-shopping habits)?

Body–mind medicine

During the time of hormonal change, our nerves are often rawer than we would like. This can happen when you are undergoing hormone replacement therapy too, even when you think the medication is working. There are situations when you lose control or are close to doing so. Unhelpful (or rude) remarks from those around you like 'pull yourself together' or 'are you freaking out again?' just make matters worse.

MINDFULNESS

An incredibly effective method for deep inner serenity and long-term balance is the practice of mindfulness. It acts like a mental airbag or safety buffer against stress. By inwardly taking a step back and looking at a situation from a distance, so to speak, you can observe your body's reactions and your feelings. This helps you to better understand what is happening to you in the particular situation.

Here's an example: my colleague gives a presentation on our joint project and doesn't mention me at all. What feelings does this evoke in me? Anger, rage, sadness, or disappointment? Do I get stomach cramps or a racing heart, or do I feel so annoyed that I can hardly breathe? Learning mindfulness also trains you to avoid making snap judgements. Could it be that my colleague did not mention my contribution to the project for a good reason? Now I come to think of it, she didn't mention her own contribution either; she just presented the facts and started off a good discussion. My pulse slows and my anger disappears.

Another example: at home my 14-year-old daughter slams the door behind her after she has given me a bolshie answer when I asked when she was planning on coming home: 'Mum, chill out, I'll see you when I see you.' I can feel my blood pressure rising, my hands get sweaty, my stomach cramps up. I hurry to the door after her, but my daughter has already disappeared into her new boyfriend's car. All I can hear is the roaring of the tuned engine as I catch a glimpse of the rear bumper. I am standing on the doorstep and grab my neck, my temples are pulsating, the lower lid of my right eye is twitching. I register my physical reaction in detail: I am so angry I could choke; the rage is pounding in my head; this child is winding me up. I know I'm allowed to react to it, but I also know that anger and fear belong to the category 'fight or flight'. I take ten deep breaths into my stomach and then I feel better. I know that I need to speak to my daughter the next day and explain that I don't want to patronise her, but that my questions stem from my concerns as her mother. My anger calms and my blood pressure is back to its normal level.

Learning mindfulness is part of body–mind medicine. Ever since treatments have been well documented by serious studies, body–mind medicine — which includes meditation and yoga as well as other stress-reduction techniques — has managed to make its way out of the esoteric corner and into the mainstream. Meditation is extremely beneficial for chronic pain (headache and back pain, for instance), high blood pressure, heart disease, chronic diseases, and is also used to great effect as an alternative therapy alongside conventional cancer treatment.

In a meta-study carried out in 2016, researchers from the University of British Colombia showed that, as a result of meditation, certain brain structures changed morphologically, that is, in their structure. Eight regions in the brain, including the frontal lobe, the hippocampus and the insular cortex were affected. These are the regions that are important for attention, memory, sensory perception, and communication between the two brain hemispheres. In a study on Buddhist monks, the University of Wisconsin had previously proven that meditation can direct brain activity towards positive feelings like compassion and kindness. For the purpose of that study, the monks' brain activity was monitored in a magnetic resonance scanner.

Currently *The ReSource Project* at the Max Planck Institute of Psychiatry, under the direction of the neuroscientist Tania Singer, is researching the influence of meditation on certain areas of the brain and the subjects of this research are also Buddhist monks.

Zindel V. Segal, Mark J. Williams, and John D. Teasdale from the University of Toronto developed advanced programs for relapse prevention in depression, which are used in psychiatry and psychosomatic therapy all over the world and which are as effective as medication. So, mindfulness-based techniques are now being used as therapies for many kinds of addiction (including addiction to alcohol, nicotine, work, eating, and sex).

Stress reduction through mindfulness is booming in medical facilities around the world and is the subject of many research projects.

The most well-known method is called mindfulness-based stress reduction (MBSR). This is a stress-reduction program, which is learned over a period of eight weeks in a group setting. MBSR was developed by the American Jon Kabat-Zinn, professor emeritus of Medicine at the University of Massachusetts. MBSR includes breathing techniques, seated meditation, and perception of bodily sensations as well as the observation of your own emotions and thoughts. One important element is the 'body scan', an exercise in which you systematically 'scan' your whole body in a recurring sequence. During a body scan, patients with chronic pain experience their body not just as a cause of pain, but their focus is also guided towards other sensations and qualities of their body. They can now perceive their body in a more complex and nuanced way and they often feel comfortable within their body at last. MBSR has a proven positive effect on the immune system and reduces stress, anxiety and pain in chronic diseases. Through various exercises, you learn how to shift down a gear and to observe your own thoughts without evaluating them or frantically clinging to them.

Jon Kabat-Zinn's underlying philosophy is: 'MBSR is an art that teaches us to look at ourselves and the world in a new, different, way and to be aware of our body, our thoughts, our feelings and perceptions.' It is about surfing on the waves of life and not sinking under them. It helps you to exercise patience because if you imagine life as a churning ocean, then you train yourself not to get caught up in the turbulence and impassability. It doesn't usually make sense to get caught up in the vortex. Mindful withdrawal as a form of MBSR can help you to steer away from the emotional chaos that is pulling you towards it. You can then look at the situation from a distance, from the outside so to speak, or at least collect your thoughts momentarily. By regaining control like this, you can develop a kind of buffer, which allows for better decision-making and reaction patterns.

Through daily mindfulness training, appropriate areas of the brain are stimulated, rather like training your muscles at the gym. At the beginning of the eight-week course, the participants are asked to set themselves some goals. At the end, they are supposed to put them aside or at least explicitly not focus on them, but instead try to focus on the moment. For many this is a completely new and surprising approach, but a very effective one. Although the goal is there, it recedes into the background and things can finally calm down. You no longer focus on future plans or past anger, but only on the moment. The only thing that matters is what is happening now. This takes away the pressure of expectation, the constant evaluation (*if I don't reach the target then I've failed*), the rush and the stress. And that alone makes everything less painful.

The exercises learned in MBSR also need to be carried out at home for an eight-week period. Being willing to spare this time — especially if you are feeling so stressed that you cannot actually spare a minute — is half the battle. The MBSR participants usually find this a challenge at first , as it tends to be the case that a stress reduction course causes more stress at first. This is normal because by definition, stressed people have the feeling that they don't have enough time, or are very literally time-poor.

These feelings change relatively quickly if you carry out the daily exercises. Your general attitude to things and, of course, to other people often becomes more relaxed. You perceive more nuances; new connections open up. You switch from 'action' mode (*I must react immediately and get angry*) into 'being' mode (*I am angry. What is happening to me right now?*). MBSR is about not judging and, instead, accepting with an open heart. Try to adopt the mindset of a curious child and see things as they are in the current moment (for example, physical sensations, emotions, sounds, and thoughts). This allows you to recognise unfavourable reaction patterns and to become more relaxed.

For example, at the beginning of the eight-week course there is an exercise that is called 'raisin meditation'. Each participant is given a raisin that they look at and feel. The participants also discuss the properties of the raisin (what type of grape did it come from, what is its country of origin, how long has it been dried for, what was it treated with). Only then may the participants put it in their mouths, chew it for what feels like an eternity, and then swallow it. A single raisin can be a real experience, even for people who don't like raisins.

The mindfulness training helps us to lose our blinkers, so that we no longer live life on autopilot and under continuous stress. You learn to recognise and curb stressful impulses that occur spontaneously. A person trained in mindfulness will, for example, be able to break through the anger that is an automatic reaction to a colleague's comment. They might ask themselves questions such as, *What is happening in my body right now? Is my heartbeat raised, are my temples pulsating, is my stomach feeling queasy? Why can a single statement upset me so much? What does this have to do with me? What does this situation remind me of?*

All feelings and all thoughts are allowed and are not evaluated or devalued. It's as though you were to freeze the scene of a movie you are watching. In the same way, a mindful person would briefly 'press the pause button' in real life and take a closer look at the situation. That way, you regain control over your own feelings and thoughts. When your brain is trained in this way, you learn to not let the flood of demands of everyday life overtake you and stress you out, but instead to pause for a brief moment and reflect. Through concentrated observation, you learn to direct your thoughts and not allow yourself to be permanently ruled by them. You decide against recurring negative thought patterns that depress your mood and cause you physical harm. Mindful behaviour enables us to look at our emotional chaos in a value-free way, and to get out of the autopilot of daily life and actively steer our lives ourselves again.

Questioning one's own value system is also part of MBSR, as is self-reflection. Do you judge others as harshly as you judge yourself? Do you judge a situation (too) quickly? How self-confident are you? Lots of people in the midlife phase don't feel as light-hearted and cheerful as they used to.

Dealing with these issues can lead to more satisfaction and a lighter mood, as can shedding any baggage. Less distraction, less hierarchy, less status, less toxic relationships, fewer clothes and possessions ... this can all be very liberating.

What do I need? In every situation where you are apprehensive, anxious or about to lose your nerve, ask yourself: what would be good for me now? What do I need right now? How can I get out of this setting for a short moment (mentally or physically) in order to gather myself? Where can I find the peace I need (lock the door behind me, sit down on the steps outside the house or in a chair in reception, go for a walk round the block or into the forest, take a hot bath, drink a cup of tea, or go to the cinema)? By taking deep breaths in and out, you can find your balance again. Often you don't have to do anything particularly special. Try whatever you find helps best. What does your 'personal airbag' involve?

The secret of stress reduction is to recognise when you are overloaded and losing your autonomy and to stop, in order to bring some space and strength back into your life. Of course, you can continue to revel in the past or you can formulate ideas for the future. The difference is that a person trained in mindfulness does it consciously.

The eight-week MBSR course discusses important questions for almost everyone interested in mindfulness: *Why don't I have any time for myself? What priority do I give to having time for myself? What does it say about my life if I can't free up 20 minutes a day for MBSR exercises? What do I want to change and how can I succeed in achieving this?* Everyone in the group learns from the answers of the others.

MBSR courses are supported by some health insurance companies — check with yours.

Of course, you won't develop a mindful attitude overnight, which is why the basic course takes two months, but it is one of the cornerstones of mindfulness training. You deal with the straitjacket of evaluation that is confining you, and with the many habits you have that hinder your personal development. You learn to recognise and overcome any awkward, threatening, and negative behaviours that you might be clinging to.

For example, we humans tend to evaluate people and situations within a few seconds. This behaviour goes way back into human history, and was an advantage for survival in terms of evolution. If you could spot from a distance that the person approaching you was coming after you, then exhibiting anger and aggression was an appropriate defence mechanism to scare the enemy away. Nowadays, it makes little sense — for example — to see all the other drivers on the road as incompetent or to take an instant dislike to your new colleague because she is wearing a skirt with a weird pattern. It takes a lot of thought and energy to overcome our prejudices and, for example, get to know the new colleague (who turns out to be really nice!). A mindful person notices the skirt and the person wearing it and accepts both of them: a patterned skirt and a woman. No more, no less.

THE PILLARS OF MINDFULNESS

Be in the here and now: observe what's going on in your body right now. Not yesterday, not tomorrow, but here and now.

Be patient: life happens in its own time. It doesn't help to rush or push things. There is no turbo-spin program for personal growth.

Allow trust: trusting in your own intuition and your own life are the best ways to relax. This also implies trust in your own body, which knows exactly what is right and wrong, and sends the corresponding warning signals.

Accept things as they are: before things can change, they have to be accepted. If I am not willing to acknowledge my pain or my burnout, if I deny my condition or conceal it from myself or others, then I cannot do anything about it. Accepting the situation is an important key to the healing process.

Don't judge; be impartial: do you sugar-coat things or avoid difficult situations? We see self-deception all around us, but it doesn't get us anywhere. In the same way, you spoil things for yourself when you jump to conclusions about people and situations. Instead, it is worth approaching people and situations in an open and honest way.

Be open to new experiences: we live in a goal-orientated era. Nothing happens without purpose. Mindfulness is about letting go of this. Let yourself be surprised, and be open to new things. It's not a bad thing to have goals, of course, but they should not dominate your life. This will make you focus too much on the future and will cause you to be less present for your life from moment to moment.

Take responsibility: take responsibility for your own life. You can achieve this by managing and reducing your expectations of others. Then you have a better chance of not being disappointed or feeling like a victim.

Learn to let go: thoughts and convictions that we cling to can exert power over us and cause illness. Mindfulness helps us to recognise what we can and must let go of, and how we can achieve this. This includes gently letting go of certain people, painful memories, and bad situations.

Mindfulness is one of the best preventative methods there is when it comes to mental and physical health. You have probably experienced times when you see things without really noticing them or eat things without really tasting them. Sometimes you might arrive somewhere in your car without remembering the journey there.

The same thing can happen with your body. Many symptoms can develop on the basis of small physical changes. In the previous chapters you discovered how the various hormones in their regulatory circuits are connected to one another. Hormone glands in the body are steered by the brain, and vice versa; everything that happens in the body is registered by the brain. But if we don't pay attention to this permanent flow of information, which affects the immune, nervous, and cardiovascular systems, the organs, all the hormones and transmitters and every single tiny little cell — if we are not focused or concentrating enough — then serious and significant health problems can develop. Which brings us back to our core belief: everything is connected to everything else. Or as Jon Kabat-Zinn says, 'The essence of training our mind in mindfulness is knowing what to do in the moment.' Mindfulness is the best guide for your 'inner doctor'.

Mindfulness does not mean that you will never encounter any more problems. But a different way of looking at things will help: each new challenge that you have to face is a call for personal growth. Everyone who has reached the middle phase of their life can look back on a wealth of experience. Life is a big, long river. Sometimes the water flows calmly, sometimes it rages, sometimes it's murky, sometimes it's clear. Existential crises, illness, love, loss, disappointments, joy, happiness, and everything else besides are the ingredients. The highs and lows of life are often the most important teachers. If you recognise this, then you can be more relaxed in dealing with the next chaos that the flow of life brings you. When the basic internal balance is right and you feel stable, you can take a step back and look at what is happening in that moment, take a deep breath, and, with composure, you can make the right decision. Overcoming obstacles makes us strong and brings us a step forward. To quote Kabat-Zinn once again, 'Only a storm-tested captain is a good captain.'

MEDITATION

Meditation is an important exercise within MBSR, but it is also a contemplative exercise in its own right. Archaeologists have found cave murals thousands of years old in Afghanistan, Pakistan, and India illustrating meditation practices. In traditional Chinese medicine, meditation is a form of therapy that strengthens the body, mind, and soul and promotes the healing process.

It is scientifically proven that regular meditation alleviates pain and strengthens the immune system. Meditation is effective in chronic illnesses, pain therapy, and depression (particularly preventing relapses). Meditation can help cancer patients adjust to their new situation and to gather their resources and strength.

You can meditate anywhere and anytime. You don't need to have a meditation cushion at hand, or to be able to sit in the lotus position, or to have much time. One of the most well-known meditation methods is transcendental meditation (referred to often as 'TM'). It was founded by the Indian teacher Maharishi Mahesh Yogi and introduced to the western world in the 1950s. In this practice, someone learning meditation is given a suitable, personal, wise mantra by their meditation teacher. They use this mantra for the meditation that they carry out twice a day in a seated position. TM belongs to the category *passive, still meditation*; in the active version, the student walks around and sings the mantras.

At least at the beginning, five minutes of sitting still on a chair is enough. Your breath should calm. You take four breaths in and eight breaths out. If you are new to meditation, you will find it is hard to sit still for much more than a second without a million thoughts coming and going through your mind: *how hard is this chair, did I switch my phone off, what time is it, can't the neighbours be quieter, I still have to buy tomatoes, I like my new colleague, but my old one is becoming more and more annoying, when are the holidays starting* ... and so on and so forth.

In order to calm your thoughts, you need to concentrate on your breath. 'I breathe in, I breathe out.' Once the breath has become automatic, then you can concentrate on a specific point. You look at the keyhole in the door, for example, if your chair is near it, or if you have your eyes closed you concentrate on the inner point between your eyes. When a thought then pops into your head, you let it pass and return to concentrating on your focus point (which at some point you will no longer notice).

Increase the time you meditate from five minutes three times a week to ten, 15, 20, then 30 minutes. You might achieve that feeling of inner peace within just a few weeks and the need to meditate regularly might become quite strong. The body and soul are inquisitive students, and they quickly learn what is good for them. Meditation 'professionals' who meditate regularly for at least half an hour in the mornings and evenings have often been practising meditation for many years.

Meditation ideally happens in quiet surroundings, whether at home or in the park, for example. You might need to communicate your need for quiet by locking the door and maybe hanging up a 'Do not disturb' sign. This way everyone knows what's going on and you know that you won't be disturbed. Of course, you need to switch off your mobile and leave your landline off the hook. But it is not all that important to have continuous quiet, and that's hardly ever possible anyway. During your meditation, you might hear the children playing outside, or the local construction site, but you will keep returning your concentration to your breath and your internal or external point of focus.

The challenge lies in the acceptance. Even if feelings of sadness, restlessness, or fear arise during meditation, you can open yourself up to them and allow them to pass, which releases pressure.

There will always be days where you can't sit still for more than five minutes or your thoughts refuse to be calm, despite years of practising. But don't let this get you down — it happens to everyone. If meditation was tricky today, you can sit down and try again tomorrow.

You quickly become aware of the positive effects of meditation. You will remain calmer in stressful situations and you will find an inner peace. You can sometimes even feel the deep muscles in your face relaxing during the meditation. Celebrities questioned about how they look so good often cite meditation and yoga as a miracle cure. Saying that meditation is all it takes for a wrinkle-free forehead is probably a lie, but nonetheless there is some truth to it.

During the time when you manage to find silence, you will get to know your mind. Which thoughts come along most frequently, which ones interest you, and what feelings and moods are created by your merry-go-round of thoughts?

At the beginning, many meditators are genuinely shocked when they find out how much time they spend in regret, in planning for the future, or clinging to the past. During the meditation practice, you become curious about which thoughts might come along. If you greet a thought with an open heart and don't evaluate or catalogue it, then this can remove a lot of the pressure. If you keep having thoughts about future obligations (*I have to do this and that*), it can make you feel restless and impatient. It can be helpful to assign a thought to a category, for example, *planning*. So, if you have another thought like ... *and I haven't got around to doing my tax returns yet either* ... often accompanied by a rapid heartbeat, then you can assign it the term *planning* and concentrate on your breath again. And this is what you do every time — regardless of which thought is trying to make itself noticed, it loses its power. It is simply just a thought like any other, which will come and go.

Thought production is a continuous process, in the same way that small children babble to themselves. Studies have shown that only about 10 per cent of all thoughts that enter our consciousness are actively thought; the rest plop into a sort of *brain digestion*. So, you don't need to act on all these thought-requests; that would be much too stressful. Think about how high the stress levels are for people who don't meditate or practise relaxation techniques!

BREATHING IS LIVING

We breathe in and out, unconsciously, around 18,000 times a day. With the in-breath, we provide all the cells in our body with fresh oxygen, while the out-breath expels used air together with a decent portion of carbon dioxide. We rarely breathe consciously, and certainly not deep into our abdomen. However, active, slow, deep breaths are the basis of all relaxation methods. 'Proper' breathing calms the autonomic nervous system, lowers our heart rate and blood pressure, and also calms our thoughts.

There are many different schools of breathing. In Ayurvedic *Pranayama*, different breathing exercises are used, such as deep breathing into the abdomen. With the in-breath, the abdomen curves outwards; with the out-breath, the abdomen automatically pulls inwards. The out-breath is supposed to be twice or three times as long as the in-breath. Counting helps: inhale up to a count of three or four, exhale to a count of by six or eight. In difficult, tense moments, you can apply this relaxing form of deep breathing and immediately notice how your entire nervous system relaxes.

Kapalabhati breathing promotes the exhalation of carbon dioxide from the lungs. You breathe in through the nose and exhale with short, powerful bursts through the mouth.

By using the alternate nostril breathing technique called *Anuloma Viloma,* the cells in the body are cleansed. You alternate the breath through each nostril. For this you place your right thumb on your right nostril and breathe in for several seconds through your left nostril. Then you hold both nostrils closed with your right thumb and right ring finger, and hold your breath for four seconds, before you open the right nostril and breathe out for twice as long again. It is key to always breathe in through the nostril that you just breathed out of, and then to switch again for the exhale. One round — right, left — repeated up to eight times. In the beginning it is quite challenging, primarily because you feel like you are going to suffocate. However, if you carry out the alternating breath on a regular basis, you will quickly see how much more breath you have and above all, how easily you can control your own breath. An evidence-based study was able to show that this alternating breath lowers blood pressure, heart rate and cortisol levels.

In particular, nasal breathing activates the parasympathetic nervous system, which acts as a stress reducer. The muscles relax and the alpha waves, an indicator for relaxation in the brain, increase. Alternate nasal breathing for 15 minutes is optimal. Learning Pranayama is worth its weight in gold.

OUR AUTONOMIC NERVOUS SYSTEM

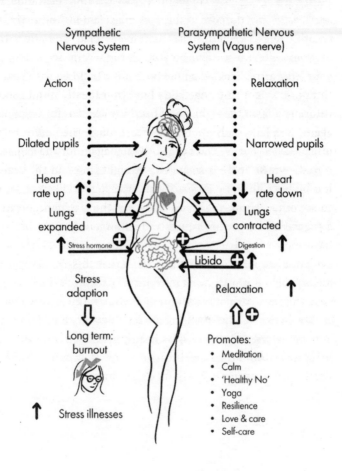

Sympathetic Nervous System

Parasympathetic Nervous System (Vagus nerve)

Action

Relaxation

Dilated pupils

Narrowed pupils

Heart rate up

Heart rate down

Lungs expanded

Lungs contracted

Stress hormone

Digestion

Libido

Stress adaption

Relaxation

Long term: burnout

Promotes:
- Meditation
- Calm
- 'Healthy No'
- Yoga
- Resilience
- Love & care
- Self-care

Stress illnesses

Balancing two antagonists

HEADING IN THE RIGHT DIRECTION

India has had its own Ministry of Yoga since 2014, and there's even an International Yoga Day, celebrated since 2015. Yoga is a recognised traditional healing method as well as a physical and mental practice. For this purpose, certain positions (asanas), breathing (pranayama), relaxation, concentration, meditation, and regeneration exercises are learned. During a yoga class, the various positions and techniques are alternated and sequenced to build on one another.

Yoga not only tones the body but also balances mind and soul. After just a few classes, you will find you are already feeling more relaxed and balanced. Meanwhile there are myriad different yoga forms: Hatha yoga, Vinyasa yoga, Bikram yoga, and Hormone yoga, to name a few. There is something for all tastes and all purses, all time budgets, and all abilities. The positive health effects are proven: among other things, yoga improves your ability to concentrate and strengthens your cardiovascular and immune systems.

Alongside yoga there are many other worthwhile relaxation techniques, such as Tai Chi and autogenic training. It doesn't matter what you start with or which method you eventually decide upon: you are on the right path, as you are finally taking time for yourself! So many courses are covered by health insurance companies now. Enquire with your company.

Relationships and sexuality

When you decide to learn mindfulness, meditation, or other relaxation techniques, you automatically set off on a journey of personal discovery. The questions posed at the beginning of this chapter grow ever more pressing the further you venture on your journey. This naturally also has implications for those around you.

Countless women — friends, acquaintances, and patients — have told us that they are trapped in a personal situation that is much more than a relationship crisis. Of course, there are numerous reasons why partnerships break up, but the hormone chaos that takes place for women is definitely difficult for everyone. That includes not only your partner but also other members of the family, your children, siblings and parents, as well as friends. Many women have learned to grit their teeth and carry on, often beyond the point where it no longer makes sense and is even unhealthy. This does not leave much space for our own feelings.

We put on a brave face in front of the children, and we try not to show any weakness in front of our colleagues or make ourselves vulnerable to criticism at work. We have learned not to comply with everything (or to accept too many awful compromises) and to be more understanding when we communicate with others. These tactics may have worked well for a time. Everyone might have been happy: partners, friends, work colleagues, bosses or, if you were the boss, employees. For many women, menopause is a time when these old patterns of behaviour no longer work, and they feel like something needs to give.

Case study: Am I a bad mother?

46-year-old Anna, who has three children, says: 'The words "mood swings" don't sound like anything serious, but to me they are. I have always considered myself a loving mother and good partner. Now I often feel like I can't cope. Even my children, whom I love dearly, get on my nerves. I feel like I am trapped in a hamster wheel and can't get any peace and quiet at home. When I want to do some admin at my desk, I find I'm constantly disturbed by my children's questions and the noise from their rooms. They might just be chatting or laughing with friends or playing the piano. I have become extremely sensitive to noise and start getting cross at the slightest little thing. Sometimes I even shout. I constantly feel that I'm treated unjustly. It is crazy, but I sometimes feel like the entire family are ganging up on me. Although I am surrounded by people all day at work, I feel lonely and misunderstood. On top of that, small things completely throw me; I regularly have a meltdown. My family thinks that I constantly misunderstand things. Of course, I read that it is normal to experience mood swings at my age, but these words don't in any way describe how terrible and desperate I feel. My husband, who was very understanding at the beginning, makes me feel like he no longer knows me. "You used to just nag us occasionally, but now you start shouting as soon as we come through the door!" he says. And do you know what? I no longer recognise myself either!'

When your hormones do their own thing, you are suddenly left in the lurch by the systems that used to work well. Of course, you shouldn't give in to every mood, and you need to be prepared to compromise when you're communicating with others. But when the hormone-triggered mood swings gain the upper hand it often becomes impossible to maintain control. Like Anna said, this sounds crazy and, for those who have never experienced it, inconceivable. But that is how it is. A harsh word from your partner, a misunderstanding among colleagues, a naïve comment from one of your children, or an unconscious slight by a friend, and you lose your cool. You notice your own 'failures' or 'shortcomings' and you want to hide, but you don't know whether that's in shame or because you are angry with yourself. The loss of control generates anger, guilt, a screaming fit, or complete silence. And infinite pressure. Of course, this pressure is hard to bear, especially in the long run.

So, take the pressure off. In our experience, open communication helps. No one will understand how you are feeling if you don't communicate. This is why we think it is imperative and helpful to talk about any difficulties you are having — perhaps not with your employer initially, but with family and friends. In order to do this, you need to know what is happening to you. The more knowledge you have, the more easily you can talk to others about this phase of your life, and the better it will be for you and those around you.

> SEB: 'I sat my husband and children down for dinner and talked to them about the fact that the whole family was currently suffering from hormone issues: three children in puberty, their mother in perimenopause, and their father at the age when most men dream about getting a motorbike. Their father was thinking about other things, as he already had the motorbike licence and the motorbike had been stolen from outside our house. This didn't make things any better ... I complained about the fact that everyone left too much mess around, they were too loud, we were too disorganised. I'm sure these things are true of all families and were no reason for me to sink into despair. But I did. Time and again. Which is why I tried to explain to my family that unfortunately, my feelings get the better of me, and I need to sort them out for myself. I think my children were grateful for this explanation, because it stopped them from feeling that they were not normal or that they had been badly behaved. The openness led to a better understanding between us all and we all felt much happier. Now, we can usually laugh things off or at least not turn them into a drama. I have learned not to be so affected by my own mood swings. And I can now see when I need some time off — which benefits all of us.'

We can't offer couples therapy here and, in any case, every relation-ship has its own rules and dynamics. One woman I interviewed for this book told me that she'd been married to at least four men over the last 20 years. But she didn't mean four different men — *just her one and only*. She had fallen in love with the student with the sexy body and long black hair, a free spirit, who had spent several years travelling the world. This man, who never wanted to stay in, who danced the night away and then drove her in his car at three in the morning to take in the sunrise on a North Sea beach with his arms around her, was by her side for three years. Then came the young professional who cut his hair, left the house in a suit, and returned home in the evenings, exhausted and often grumpy. Instead of going to clubs, he now hit the tennis court, went jogging in the park, went to the cinema, or straight to bed. She then swapped this guy for the father of her four children, who took on the role of a house-husband for several years and did a great job. During this time, she never saw him wearing a suit; he now had very short hair and a hipster beard. He made breakfast for the family wearing the white T-shirt he had slept in. When she returned home in the evenings, he waved to her contentedly from the terrace. And for some years now she's been married to a project manager who is responsible for the construction of industrial plants all over the world. When he returns from business trips that last several weeks, he talks animatedly of his impressions of other cultures, and he even smells different when she greets him at the airport. Smells from India, Asia, or Africa are still on his clothes and head. He no longer has any hair.

When we are in a long-term relationship, we naturally go through different phases of life. Life is change, whether we like it or not. As my interviewee made clear in our open conversation, of course, it's not only women who change, but men too. And yes, hormones are partially responsible for this as well. But still, it's lovely to see someone falling in love with the same man time and again, even though he comes in three or four different forms over the years. How refreshing to look at the other person with new eyes and a keen interest and allow him the space to make these changes for himself. How wonderful to enjoy the newly won insights in each phase of life together with your partner.

If we were all lucky and able enough to do this, we would surely all live in tolerant, happy relationships that are never boring. We would always be interested in the other person; we'd always find them desirable and sexy. Unfortunately, in reality it's not so easy. That just doesn't happen in most relationships (or most bedrooms).

Life goes through phases. For a while childcare takes up most of your attention, or perhaps yours or your partner's career is at the forefront. What do you do with your all your free time once the children have moved out or you retire? What do you have to say to each other when you are not talking about everyday stuff and the children, the house, your hobbies, organising your next holiday, and visits to the extended family? These are new, unfamiliar situations that affect both partners and that need to be discussed together. We encourage you to do that. It's great if you can speak to each other lovingly and discuss your ideas and hopes in an open way. This requires honesty and is often the vital ingredient for the success of many more years together. Expectations of relationships and friendships change and in most women, these are further intensified by the hormonal changes we go through. Our nerves might be frazzled, we might be less patient, or more easily offended. We might feel criticised, misunderstood, or ignored. Chances are, we are no longer prepared to put up with a lot of the things that we let our partner get away with over the years or that have become a habit. We tend to expect greater respect than we used to. And of course, this works both ways.

Thinking about your own role and eventually deciding that you no longer want to be seen as just a mother, wife, sexual partner or family provider changes everything. Something very paradoxical happens, because as you discard this role, your personality deepens. Many women report that they long for something else in their life. Many become more open to exploring spirituality. In order to avoid unnecessary conflict, you should talk to your family about the way you are feeling. This prevents disparaging remarks based on ignorance, which you really don't need right now.

Long-smouldering conflicts or frustrations in a relationship can surface when children grow up. This is known as empty-nest syndrome. Looking after the children is no longer at the forefront and couples need to focus their attention on their own relationship again. This often raises the question of how much of it is left after all these years. Both partners have to think about this both separately and together. When each person takes stock of themselves, the result of their new self-knowledge can be surprising for their partner. As a result, this is a time when relationships often change — especially if one partner realises that their own needs have not been met for many years, and perhaps never will be met in this relationship. Couples therapists are inundated with partners going through the midlife phase. Many people experience a change in their need for closeness and sexuality and this can become a huge issue for the relationship.

SEXUALITY

During menopause, sex is the last thing many women are thinking of. The idea of actively seducing your partner, or if you're single, dating or masturbating, often seems downright absurd. You may be able to just about muster the energy to watch Netflix in the evenings, but even then, you tend to fall asleep. When you have used up all your energy on your daily tasks and chores, and you finally fall into bed at the end of the day, exhausted, then all you want is to be left alone. Sexual overtures from a partner would not be welcome. For those who used to really enjoy sex, this can come as a bit of a shock. Who would have thought things would change so much?

But is the general decline in sexual activity due to reduced sexual arousal, or a relationship pattern that has grown a bit stale? It has been shown that for most couples who have been married for many years, sex during the middle years is no longer central, but instead the relationship adapts to this new phase of life. However, it very much depends on the habits and behaviours that have been fostered in the relationship; there are couples who still enjoy frequent sex even after 30 years together.

During menopause, a woman's physical needs change. They are scaled back in favour of a phase of inner reflection. You may want to focus on other things, on your secret desires and new ways of expressing your personality. You often hear women who have taken a different path say, 'This is more satisfying than any partner or lover.' That can be the case — but it doesn't have to be. They are not mutually exclusive; you can be passionate about spiritual matters, for example, and still be interested in sex.

Take a bold look at your sexual needs. Do you still feel desire and, if so, are your desires being met or have you been able to fulfil them yourself over the last few years? For those who have recently fallen in love, the days seem long as they look forward to the next time they will see their new partner. But how can sexual relationships between couples who have been together for a long time be revitalised? How do you feel about your own body? Do you feel desirable? How is your self-esteem?

If society persuades older women to think they are no longer desirable or beautiful, this can nip sexual desire in the bud completely. When a hormone imbalance is making a woman feel ill, or if she is stressed or depressed, clearly this will also have a significant impact on her libido.

We know — and this isn't only through research — that women's sexuality is a complex matter. Women's desire works differently from that of men. Women react less to optical stimuli. A man's physique or appearance can be sexy but that's not always necessary for women. Feeling cared for, hearing expressions of love, and having an attentive partner ... it may sound like a cliché, but these factors can increase female desire. If women are not stimulated on an emotional and spiritual level, then not much is likely to be happen on a physical level either. Whether a woman's sex life is fulfilling depends on many factors: sex education, self-image, age, cultural background, good and bad experiences, general health, and any kind of ongoing pain (which in the case of vaginal pain could occur because of dryness due to lack of oestrogen).

Of course, a partner's empathy and the quality of the relationship in general play a decisive role. That is, perhaps, one reason the Viagra pill for women — to increase sexual desire — was such a failure. Female sexuality is too complex to be switched on and off with a pill, not to mention the side-effects.

Studies have shown that a fulfilling love life does not depend on age so much as on a woman's health. If a woman is in good health, then there should be nothing standing in the way of good sex. This is why it is so important to take care of your own health if you want a fulfilling sex life.

What we can all do without are the exhausting comparisons between ourselves and other women; comparisons that leave us feeling inadequate because we don't fit the slender, youthful ideal. This causes stress. All those associations that are related to getting older, for example the notion of being 'past your best' can be incredibly stress-inducing. These psychological factors lead to sexual problems in many women, without there being a physical cause.

Older women who are in relationships in which they feel secure and valued often have a particularly good sex life. There is no reason this shouldn't continue into old age. Women in perimenopause and menopause today feel significantly younger than previous generations did. They are often more educated about sex and also more open to experimenting — not least because the risk of an unwanted pregnancy is much reduced. This means that women can enjoy sex more openly and without fear. Many women report that this freedom and also their acceptance of their own body in this phase of life leads to an unprecedented sexual curiosity. All of a sudden, they dare to express their desires and try out things that previously only took place in their imagination. And yes, they feel desirable and sexy.

We would also like to talk about sensuality. You discover beauty in small things, breathe in the smell of herbs or a new favourite perfume, and sharpen your senses. Feeling, smelling, tasting, and touching stimulate the reward system and ensure the distribution of, among other things, dopamine and oxytocin. The rediscovery of sensuality in everyday life can be a way to reach more erotic sensuality. Like erotic massages, a foot, neck, and back Thai massage, for example, has been shown to raise oxytocin, strengthen the immune system, and lead to relaxation.

It can also make sense to have your testosterone or its precursor, DHEA, measured. It is not only in men that a lack of testosterone can dampen desire.

As we said earlier, some women do go off sex. They can't bear the thought of it; the most they might want is some physical closeness with no expectation of sex. This might be a cause of tension with their partner, and some women don't even want any physical contact at all. It's totally natural and okay to experience these different phases; at the start of perimenopause there is an increase in desire but later on the libido decreases, though this may not present any problem provided your partner is compassionate and patient. The best thing to do is to communicate that the way you're feeling is due to the stage of life you're in. If a partner is understanding, it may help a woman to feel some desire again.

For a healthy, fulfilling sexuality, it's essential to feel good about your own body. Women have been conditioned by society to be hypercritical of themselves. During menopause this tendency can intensify rather than improve. The body changes, skin becomes more sensitive and wrinkled, breasts begin to droop, and the thighs are not as firm as they used to be. Those who have always defined themselves as sexually attractive exclusively or predominantly through their appearance will fight tooth and nail against these changes. They will find it difficult. Especially in today's world of Instagram models and social media, women are under a lot of pressure to present an attractive image. For the selfie or the photo you are posting, you feel you have to look immaculate, your hair must be perfectly styled, your skin wrinkle-free — any hint of a fat roll on your tummy is a no-no. Photoshop will iron out anything that needs to go.

The human body is not perfect — no one is. To recognise the truth of this, it is worth looking at the makeover 'before and after' images of famous models. Sometimes the difference is quite incredible, and you would think that in real life, a lot of the supermodels are no more remarkable or attractive than any other woman.

Fortunately, most women who find themselves in this phase of life say that when you're in your mid-forties or mid-fifties, you worry less about what your body looks like than when you were in your mid-twenties or mid-thirties. You've finally made friends with your body; you know what it's like and how to emphasise the bits you like, and embrace, accept, or ignore the others. Sex becomes more unconstrained — you just want to have fun and find fulfilment and satisfaction. You have learned about what pleasures you, and know how to get it for yourself or ask for it from your partner. This is wonderful for your health because during an orgasm, the tissues of the vagina, uterus, and ovaries are supplied with extra blood. Moreover, there's no question that the feelings we get from a loving touch, whether given to ourselves or received from someone else, make us happy and enrich our lives. Enjoyable, sensual touch ensures that we feel loved and safe.

SEB: 'A friend of mine told me that she considers sex beneficial to health. She spoke to her friends about needing to keep just as fit "down below" as elsewhere. If she didn't have regular sex, she would be less interested in it. Regular sexual activity, which took a bit of effort from her in the beginning, had got her relationship going again.'

A healthy relationship with your own sexuality is beneficial to health, both physically and psychologically. We would like to suggest that you try masturbation if you are single or if sex with your partner does not currently give you an orgasm, or simply for the physical pleasure. By doing this you remain in touch with your body in a very personal way as it changes during menopause. This is about knowing your erogenous zones as well as knowing how to bring yourself to orgasm. Pleasing yourself is good for you.

SETTING BOUNDARIES — TURNING OFF THE ENERGY PREDATORS

Speaking of relationships, we'd like to go into toxic relationships and people who sap your energy. Nothing uses up as much energy as people who don't notice that they are constantly crossing a line, making exorbitant demands, or talking non-stop about themselves and their problems. If you were to seek advice from one of these 'energy sappers', you would probably be fobbed off and let down. This is not only unfair — it should also make you think. During phases of hormonal upheaval, you are more sensitive and more prone to disappointment. Which of us has not seen friendships fall apart when things are not going so well? Almost every woman in her middle years has seen this happen. And it raises questions: which friends shall we take with us into the next ten years? Who is still on board, who is just tolerated, who has abandoned ship, and who would you like to chuck over the rails? Who takes up too much of our energy, which we now need more than ever?

Each of us has only a limited amount of energy to use for others. If you are drained, you are of no use to anyone, and especially not to those whom you genuinely want to support with all your strength. Setting boundaries is not easy, especially if you want to be popular —and it sure isn't easy when your guilty conscience gets you with the evil word 'egotist'. You don't want to be rude; you don't want to offend. You want to keep all your options open, stay friendly and popular so that you get invited to the next social gathering. But still, at times when you have less energy, when your hormones are taking their toll, it makes sense to set boundaries and say no. You should no longer put up with relationships that have been sapping your energy for decades. Saying no can actually be very liberating.

Saying no can also come in the form of a spatial, temporal, or emotional retreat. A pleasant location, a sofa, a room where you can close the door, a favourite place outside like a lake or under a tree, or a particular park bench are great possibilities for places where you can go when everything becomes too much for you, where you can refuel for several minutes or hours.

You need to practise time management, especially as far as work is concerned. You might sometimes have to do overtime when things are very busy, but it should not become a daily habit. That will just bring you to the brink of burnout. However, time management can be applied to challenging personal situations too. It's fine to listen to your girlfriend's problems for half an hour or even a whole hour, but two hours at a time on a regular basis is definitely too much.

In principle, you should not expose yourself to draining situations. You should seek help to put a stop to any situation in which you are being harassed (which is a criminal offence). And do limit your visits to any relatives who leave you feeling bad or uncomfortable.

Case study: perimenopause and toxic relationships

Julia was a 53-year-old physiotherapist, divorced with two daughters. She had been off work for six months with burnout, was having depressive episodes, and was currently undergoing psychotherapy. Through her job, she had regularly encountered people with stress-related back problems and was also interested in holistic medicine. This made her decide to become actively involved in her own recovery. With the help of her therapist, she analysed various situations in her life where she had reacted with recurring behavioural patterns. This included recent events, a divorce, a difficult relationship with her mother, and huge pressures at work. All this had taken its toll on her. After holding everything together for years and organising her daily life as a single mother as best she could, there came a time when she had reached a low point both physically and mentally. Her life had manoeuvred her into a burnout. Julia had always seen herself as a fun-loving, active woman, and now she wanted to do everything possible to become 'the old Julia' again. With surprising openness and with help from her psychotherapist, she began to analyse the conflicts that had been simmering for years.

The call from a long-time friend was the final straw. After not having contacted her for months, the friend now poured out all her own problems at work and in her marriage, and then gave a detailed description of the holiday house she had recently bought. She didn't ask how Julia was. When Julia tried to get a word in, the friend ended the call, saying she really needed to head off to pick up her children from sports. That was the moment Julia realised that she would no longer be available for this friend.

In their midlife, women often break old patterns. They look at past and current relationships in a new light. This leads to a *shift* in the way they see friendships. Unhealthy relationships and those that are no longer working at this time of life are often radically abandoned. This is unlikely to be down to one clumsy phone call but rather to countless little unspoken things like assaults on your self-esteem, misunderstandings, and multiple other infringements. All of this, coupled with a lack of the energy you need to handle it, can lead to a healthy kind of selfishness and a clear decision: 'That's enough!'

If your parents are still alive and present in your life, even your relationship with them might change at this time. You need boundaries. After all, you are a middle-aged adult now!

It always comes down to saying 'no' in one way or another. This will require a lot of effort and strength in the beginning, but it's worth it. Saying no does not need to be rude — it can be done in a friendly manner: 'Today doesn't work for me ... maybe next time ... I already have plans ... I can't talk right now ...' Avoidance is another tactic. It means you do not even put yourself in the situation — for example, you don't offer to be a dog-sitter or babysitter or host. You might do it again some time, but not when it's going to rob you of the energy you so badly need right now.

Saying no also works within the family. Children can learn that there are times you are available for questions and discussions, and times you don't want to be disturbed or spoken to. Partners, too, should respect the fact that you are not available round the clock, but that you also need some hours off in your own space. And that might mean going to your own private room, or leaving the house for a little while.

RECHARGING

Do you ever get to the point when you completely lose it? When you holler, 'That's it, I'm leaving, I'm going to the end of the world and never coming back!'? This means your energy levels are down to zero, perhaps because you're currently going through an intensely difficult time or because you've just been through a long period of stress.

Experience has shown that during stressful phases in life, problems rarely come alone. You might be pulling your hair out or crying into your pillow at night and wishing for some magic to happen that makes everything all right by morning. But unfortunately, it's up to you. You just have to get up and carry on.

But how, when your reserves are utterly depleted?

Even if it sounds completely paradoxical, the fact is that in crisis situations, you are able to mobilise particularly powerful resources. These are mostly released in the fear and panic that a hopeless situation creates, and you are not even aware of them. Time runs away with you, you are about to move out of your flat and the boxes have not been packed yet; you just lost your job; you've been diagnosed with a serious illness; your partner left you or you are leaving them, and who knows what dark clouds loom on the horizon. You are not getting any younger ...

STOP!

In life, none of us can avoid having to navigate the impassable forest of painful emotions like suffering, disappointment, grief, and frustration. The effort is exhausting and scary. The only thing that helps is to pause, breathe, and keep your thoughts in the here and now.

In the novel *Momo* by Michael Ende, a street sweeper, Beppo, explains the secret of how to achieve an insurmountable task to the little girl Momo: one breath, one stroke of the broom, one breath, one stroke of the broom ... and eventually, you've managed the infinitely long road ahead. Along the way you think: 'I'm never going to manage this; how can I possibly do it?' Even before you've taken the first step, you are thinking about giving up.

But as we said, you won't need your special powers for ever. If you dare or force yourself to take the first step, then the second one will be easier, and all the rest even easier, until one day you reach the end of the rainbow.

At best, we will have looked at our resources and filled up with positive energy in calm, good times. Then we will be better able to respond and fall back on them when we are in a crisis situation.

However, most people are not well prepared — that is only human. It is only when the big questions in life arise — an illness, a bereavement, a crisis that becomes existential and requires decisions that go beyond the everyday — that many people wake up. Often these are crossroads in life: do I go left or right?

Interestingly, it is these difficult, hopeless situations that allow us to mature, and that can lead to a profound change in our attitude and actions. Unfortunately, we usually only realise this in retrospect.

With many women, painful dilemmas or silent goodbyes come along in parallel to the hormonal changes they are undergoing. This leads to disappointment, anger and sometimes deep sadness. This phase in which female fertility ends permanently is also a time of saying goodbye. And goodbyes need to be recognised and mourned. This process is healthy and needs time.

Ending old ways of being or toxic relationships opens up new opportunities in the long term. These gaps provide time and space and the chance for something new. If your jam-packed everyday life has had a hold on you for years, you might now be facing a cleared-out blank space. You can see this as scary, or as a great opportunity for creativity, new feelings, and a new perspective. You can paint the space royal blue, deep green or pillar-box red and also refurnish it. By the time they reach 40, women usually know what they want and what they are not prepared to put up with anymore. This is hard won, from experience. Relationship work has and is being done and personal value systems are being questioned and trained in ways we may not recognise. This also includes using your energy wisely.

CAUSE OF EXHAUSTION

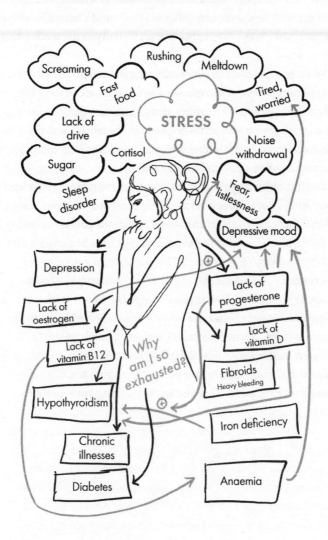

RECOGNISE YOUR OWN PERFORMANCE

Just sit back for ten minutes and think back, for example, to yesterday. What did you do, achieve, or finish? We don't just mean work-related responsibilities, but also those related to your personal life, family, friends, and neighbours. That might actually add up to quite a lot of things — possibly so much that you are astonished.

> SKB: 'In a phase of complete exhaustion, I took a pen and paper and wrote down everything I had done over the last few days. EVERYTHING: tied my son's shoelaces every morning, put together his lunch box, made his breakfast to take to nursery, took him to nursery and picked him up again later, drove to the supermarket four times, watered the plants on the balcony, started to write two articles, did three hours of internet research, read a non-fiction book and two trade journals, held three work-related telephone conversations, called my parents, made a medical appointment, organised a dinner with friends for the weekend, went to the park with my child and took the dog to the vet, did five bank transfers, cooked dinner, filled, emptied, and switched on the dishwasher three times, read 100 pages of Harry Potter to my child, washed my hair, listened to my husband for six hours, had sex, walked the dog for four hours, etc. I filled the front and back of an A4 sheet of paper, in small handwriting, written close together. I stared at this list in astonishment — it really shocked me. I think I counted close to 100 things. I am not telling you this to make my life sound more meaningful than it is or to boast about all the things that I fit into my day. On the contrary, I thought: *four supermarket visits, how badly organised am I? And how much time does the dog "cost" me? I can't believe it.* But I quickly pushed aside my immediate feelings of frustration. Instead, I turned my attention to the fact that, in combination with my hormonal chaos, my daily life was way too full and so it

wasn't surprising that I was exhausted. But most importantly, I finally saw what I was actually accomplishing. Regardless of whether others might argue that shopping is not actually work or whether I should have even included listening to my husband talk about his problems at work — it all counted to me, as it was my time I was giving up.'

Once you've made your own list, either in your head or on paper, then give yourself a pat on the back — even if no one else does.

One of the secrets of perimenopause is not to wait. Many women report that they have escaped from the vicious cycle of waiting; of expectation followed by disappointment. No one took the rubbish out? This is annoying but asking someone to do it and then getting cross afterwards is even more tiring. So, the rubbish can either stay in the bin until someone notices the smell, or you can grab it and take it out without resentment. Your partner was going to take the car to the mechanic but it's still in the driveway? Okay, then it's just going to stay there, and everyone will have to use public transport or walk. Or, if you don't want to be without it yourself, then quickly take the car to the mechanic. But without resentment.

At some point, you need to put aside power struggles, as in: 'You didn't do x, y or z, but I did ...' They are the biggest energy-guzzler and also the cause of everlasting disappointments. Why, you ask yourself in the midlife phase, should you be going through trench warfare? Life is too good, too short, too exciting. Better to get right into action, into doing. But if you are already doing too much, what then?

Delegate, let go is our suggestion.

DELEGATE, LET GO

When something is bothering you, try to let it go. When you have too much going on, you have to drop things or pass them on. If you want others to do them, you have to *delegate*. But what do you need to let go of? And how does it work?

In times of upheaval, when we feel we have no control over our life and we're on a constant treadmill, many of us lose touch with ourselves. The deep relationship with our inner self is overlaid by constraints, responsibilities, work, stress, media consumption, and much more.

> SEB: 'One patient reported feeling she had to juggle so many aspects of her life that having to concentrate on not dropping anything completely stressed her out. Of course, the demands on her also included things she had chosen, like professional success, doing a good job of raising her children, maintaining friendships, and also the wish, as a grown woman, to be a "good" daughter.'

This leads us to the subject of letting go, because, for example, you should not be taking on the role of mother to your parents! You are the mother of your children and the daughter of your parents, full stop. In many families the expectations between generations carry a huge potential for stress.

Letting go means dropping all those things that you don't feel are essential to you as a person. In spiritual terms, it's about the 'ego'. This can be a position, an area in which you live, a hobby without which you don't feel you can socialise, a relationship ... The list is endless.

But what do you really need and what gives you strength, rather than just using up your energy? Who or what are you angry with and therefore stressed out by? What things make you chase your tail and feel that you can't be yourself (for example, when you rush from one social engagement to the next without being able to actually enjoy yourself, and all you do is gossip about people afterwards)?

How did you end up being the person you never wanted to be? Or perhaps you've become the person you wanted to be but realise that this costs far too much energy. (There would be no blame attached to this — it's an incredibly honest and healthy insight!)

Letting go is a process of listening to yourself. You recognise yourself through honest answers. Some people in perimenopause are in a phase in their lives where they have almost everything. If you are one of these privileged people, you don't need to prove yourself anymore, you have a lot of things in the material sense and have seen some of the world. If you can't start letting go now, then will you ever be able to do it?

80 PER CENT IS GOOD ENOUGH

Those who feel totally comfortable in their value system and in their daily lives, but who are in danger of collapsing under overly high expectations, may be suffering the effects of their own perfectionist aspirations. If you've been feeling for ages that every day is too short, you have to keep giving it your all, you have to do everything right to keep things going, and woe betide if you don't, then this 'turbo gear' won't keep working for long. The more tasks you burden yourself with, the more rushed and discontented you will be. Many women push themselves to the limit in the belief that the good life requires complete focus on every front. Working overtime, taking an online course, working out in the mornings before work, trying out the latest diet fad, attending events out of some kind of fear of missing out rather than actual desire, feeling pressure to buy new clothes or to spend money on things that will 'keep up appearances', or spending an unbearable amount of time keeping your home looking neat and tidy. Who is responsible for this image of superwoman, and how long are we going to keep chasing our own tail? Is it really necessary? Who does this behaviour serve?

Thanks to the patriarchal culture we live in, women tend towards perfectionism because they often believe that it's only when you completely devote yourself to a cause that you will be loved and given the recognition you long for. We can't offer an in-depth psychological interpretation of the pursuit of perfection here, but we will say is that nobody is a failure or less valuable as a human being if they are not perfect.

If, as a perfectionist, you can allow yourself to believe this just a little bit, this will reduce a lot of pressure and alleviate physical symptoms like tension and anxiety. It also takes away the fear of making mistakes and ensures that things get done. Perfectionists often struggle to 'see things through' because their standards are so high that the project or task logically cannot be completed because it is never perfect.

For creatives, such as architects and artists, perfectionism can sometimes be a motivating force that allows them to lose themselves and create amazing things. So, perfectionism in itself is not necessarily harmful. But for a lot of people, perfectionism causes nothing but suffering.

If, like many women, you are prone to perfectionism, then make your own decision: which things give you joy and fulfil you, and which ones cost you time and nervous energy without much reward?

SEB: 'During my years abroad, I often met women who were amused by the mentality of German women. We have some strange idea that we have to do everything ourselves. Some women even clean up their flat and perhaps even polish the shower after the cleaner has been (those who have the luxury of a cleaner). I think my French friend has the right idea. She is an intellectual, successful career woman, and a mother. And a terrible home-maker. I get inspired by our evenings together. We don't only talk about the latest trends in home decor (we are not interior designers) or our children's academic performance. We talk about everything under the sun and we just enjoy ourselves. Naturally, cracked plates and un-ironed tablecloths are part of the deal.

'I remember throwing big parties and driving myself up the wall with the preparations. Every detail had to be perfect. As a result, I would be feeling very tense, which often led to big family rows just before the guests arrived. In retrospect, I can laugh at myself. It was all unnecessary and I'd brought it on myself. Nobody noticed the tablecloth I had hurriedly purchased (my 17th), which was the famous last straw that broke the camel's back.

'These days I give everyone a task. What happens is no longer solely my responsibility. Sometimes things can just be low-key. During the time we spend with our loved ones, it is the moments of closeness, the genuine interaction with the other person that remains memorable. Don't destroy that with mistaken priorities and demands. And definitely don't wear yourself out, either!'

It's worth considering which areas of your life you could spend less effort on. You can see it as your personal *energy-conservation program*. A little effort and energy saved here and there will result in disproportionately good results. When the pressure is off, the pleasure returns.

Hand things over, and remember, it's not shameful to get help. Sometimes getting just ten minutes more for yourself can allow you to replenish your reserves with this *quality time*.

Mothers are often torn between personal commitment and the fear of being a bad parent. For many of us, this motherhood guilt has been passed down from generation to generation. Although the struggle for equal rights continues, many women now experience more equality in their parenting arrangements than previous generations did. And yet, this guilt often hangs around. When it comes to your children, as in other areas, letting go can be crucial to your health (which can, in turn, benefit their wellbeing). It takes a village to raise a child, so reach out to whatever support you can access, and remember that everyone who cares for and educates your child is sharing the load of raising them. You can organise and call on help and support.

There are so many things you can delegate without having to feel bad. By grade three at the latest, your kids might be able to make their own way to class by bike, bus, or train, and this might help to build their resilience and self-confidence. Most teenagers can tidy their own rooms, and it's time they did. You can find a professional to file your tax returns, even if it feels like a huge investment initially. In fact, delegating these tedious things saves most people a lot of trouble, time, and money. Passing on professional and personal tasks is not lazy — it creates some space, which can benefit your health, no matter how you use it. In executive circles, delegating is considered a leadership quality.

People who cannot or do not yet want to delegate might come around to it eventually, creating time for themselves in their own way. We are not telling you what to do, just suggesting some ideas.

Thanks to Marie Kondo, minimalism and organisation have been a hot topic for a number of years now. We used to call it 'tidying up your room', and now we call it *life-changing magic* or *decluttering*. It is not only our work desks that are overflowing, but also, at some point, it's cellars, lofts, garages, wardrobes, and drawers. If you don't move house on a regular basis and get forced to sort through your things, then it's perfectly normal to still have many of your past possessions (from the first citrus juicer that you bought yourself as a student, which is lying in a box somewhere in the cellar, to the nice shoes you bought with your first pay cheque). But when did you actually last miss these items, or use them and, more importantly: when will you use them again? If you're totally honest, the answer may well be, never. Objects that don't have any emotional memory value can be passed on, sold, or thrown away. Yes, you can do it — it won't hurt, and it will create space, time (you won't need to shift ten boxes around anymore whenever you need something from the one at the bottom), and freedom. You won't need to make any big decisions, pack your suitcase for hours on end, or pay the extra charge for excess baggage. Having a clear-out has a lot of benefits: you go through life more lightly.

REST PERIOD = PERSONAL TIME OFF

Once you've got rid of toxic relationships, set boundaries, and learned to say no, worked on and let go of certain things that stress you out, decluttered your home and delegated a few things in your daily life, then you can embrace a long-lost friend: time.

> SKB: 'I am standing on the edge of a green, lush meadow on a beautiful late summer's day and take off my shoes. I run across the grass and hop around like a little girl. I pick a bouquet of dandelions, clovers, juniper branches on the edge of the meadow, or a cherry or plum from a tree. Then I lie down in the meadow, put the cherry in my mouth, notice how the red juice runs down my chin, wipe the drops off with the back of my hand, and clasp my hands behind my head. I blink up at the sun and there isn't a cloud in the sky. Maybe a bird chirps or a sheep bleats somewhere in the distance. This is what unplanned time feels like to me — free and calm. How do you picture it?'

The thought of having time to yourself is a kind of mirage for many women entering perimenopause. You might be afraid it will disappear as soon as you get within a few feet of it. That's how long you might have been in the desert.

Rest time is exactly what the name implies: rest. Whether you are sitting in an armchair and looking out through the window, lying in bed and listening to your favourite song 30 times over, or in the bath, topping up the hot water because you just don't want to get out — whatever you decide on each day, you are allowed to spend your free time however you want. No obligations, and you don't owe anyone an explanation — even if it requires drastic measures to defend this rest period. If necessary, lock the bathroom door, and ignore the calls and knocks. Provided you've asked if anyone needs to use the bathroom first, no one needs to come in. In the same way that nobody needs to come into your bedroom to fetch something once you've sat down on your meditation cushion, the bedroom can also be used as a place of rest during the day.

In our experience, women need a bit more practice to give themselves permission to do all those things we discussed in this chapter. This seems to be a typical feminine trait, whose roots are deeply embedded in our gendered culture and the way we are educated and socialised. At the risk of using a cliché, few men consciously or unconsciously ask permission. They simply do what they want and often only address the consequences when they are met with criticism or resistance. And that doesn't often happen. How nice for them! Women anticipate what might happen if they allow themselves something, and what consequences they might have to reckon with, especially on an emotional level. This kind of unconscious feeling of holding back will ebb away the more often you have your rest time and 'me time'. Then joy and pleasure set in and, with them, the healing and preventative processes that so benefit your health. Self-compassion is the prerequisite for taking your own needs seriously and taking the steps you need to be healthy.

Change your view of yourself: self-compassion

What do you think about yourself? That is one of the essential questions on the way to fulfilment, harmony and happiness. Even if the answer is: 'I'm an ugly little duckling and I've done everything wrong in my life,' you're on the right path simply because you're thinking about it.

When we talk about self-compassion and self-love, we can't avoid dealing with the opposite: fear, shame, anger, imperfection, lack of self-worth, weaknesses, and so on. These are the big issues that need to be looked at, which will open the door to inner balance, a healthy self-esteem, and healing. People who by virtue of their profession are intensely involved with the whole range of human feelings cannot avoid regularly looking deep into their own psyche.

SEB: 'During my training as an MBSR teacher, I attended a workshop together with 30 psychologists, psychiatrists, doctors, teachers, and people from other social professions. All of them had qualifications gained through their studies and their practice, so they had years of experience in dealing with the human psyche and were familiar with the practice of mindfulness. At the end of the course, following a long meditation exercise, everyone was supposed to write down their biggest fear on a piece a paper. We had dealt with the topic of fear a lot over the previous days. When everyone had finished writing everything down, we sat in a large circle on our meditation cushions. You could have heard a pin drop. One person after another read their sentence out loud: "I am frightened of not being good enough, that my efforts won't be enough, that I won't be able to make it, that I will fail, that I have no faith in myself, that others think I am just putting on a front ..." Interestingly, no one feared a terrible disease, losing someone, or a financial loss. Every single one of them was afraid of not being not good enough, being imperfect, or failing. This deep human fear united everyone in the room. This realisation had something immensely healing and comforting about it. It really touched me, and I will always remember that moment.'

These and other feelings of doubt, which make you question yourself, hold the greatest chance for inner growth. If we look at our weaknesses and learn to live with them, then we will overcome the state of rigidity and paralysis (*that's the way I am, I can't do anything about it, I hide behind my shame*) and become more active. Often it is the weaknesses that make us lovable and unique. We are more complex, contradictory, and paradoxical than we think. We are also more excited, more vulnerable, and less cool. Over the years we may have acquired a particular role or developed a protective shell, but underneath we are unparalleled. Not having to hide your true self behind a façade can be an extreme relief, and therefore reduces stress.

In working life, you have to be professional in your appearance and behaviour, which can be demanding enough in itself. But you usually behave the way people expect you to among friends, too. You are either the sporty one, the hostess, the generous one, the brave one, the miserly one, the sensitive one, the cheerful one, and so on. As time goes on, you merge with this version of yourself.

If you're not in a good mood, you hide your sadness or grumpiness as soon as you run into friends, even if it's only to avoid lengthy explanations ('This isn't like you, what's up?'). You deceive others, but also yourself. You like to think that you are generous, tolerant, reliable, and loving. But are you always? Fortunately, we humans are not robots, and that is why we will (hopefully) continue to be superior to artificial intelligence in emotional matters. We have so many different feelings — love, jealousy, longing, passion, joy. It is no surprise that the stories that most reflect our heart and soul are the ones that move us in literature and films.

Self-compassion begins with contemplating one's own feelings — the good and the bad. It is important to look at them in a clear and unembellished way. And it's hard because honesty, especially with regard to weaknesses and uncertainties, is not always rewarded in our society. We tend to evaluate and judge far too quickly. If we need to permanently suppress a character trait that defines us, this can lead to emotional pain, low moods, and depression. In order to avoid this trap into which so many people fall or in which they are stuck for so many years, we should show ourselves the same compassion we give our children, partners, parents, or friends.

We give ourselves such a hard time. If an evaluation of our work was poor, we call ourselves 'failures'; if we didn't get that freelance commission, we 'weren't good enough'. If we panic during turbulence on a flight, then we are 'not in control'. A fairer and gentler approach towards ourselves would serve us well. If you can't get out of bed on a Saturday morning although you should have gone grocery shopping, mowed the lawn, written an article, and called your mother, then you are not a lazy person. It's the weekend, why should you have to set an alarm? What is your guilty conscience achieving here? Nothing! Instead, you should turn over again in your bed. When you phone your mother later, you will have slept well and be in a good mood. The neighbour's lawnmower is humming; maybe she will offer to mow your lawn too. It doesn't cost anything to ask. You can send your teenagers off to do the shopping — that sounds like a great idea. All the great things you can learn about self-compassion on a Saturday morning!

Most of us are less kind to ourselves than we are to others. And those who are habitually too hard on themselves feel imperfect and unloved. This creates a vicious cycle: those people who don't feel loved crave external recognition. If this doesn't happen immediately, it is followed by frustration, shame, or withdrawal. People isolate themselves because they feel unloved and unlovable. If I admire and praise others, but criticise myself for every little thing, belittling and condemning myself, then I put up an artificial wall between myself and others. Many women who have been doing this for many years say they see themselves differently from the way they are perceived by others. Self-compassion, that is, being more forgiving and kind with yourself, can lead us out of there. We learn to understand and not to judge.

Let's be clear: we are not talking about self-pity. Self-compassion has a different quality. It helps you recognise not only the difficult circumstances you might be in, but also your years of effort and struggle. What do you think you need to be ashamed of, what is the cause of your permanent unhappiness, which characteristics do you perceive as painful, what did you think you needed to endure, is your value system in alignment with how you actually think and feel? By addressing these questions in a loving, caring way, you take on responsibility for yourself. Finding answers that work for you — not for others — allows you to grow. There is space again in your life for you to feel good about yourself, happy, and mentally and physically stable — which is how it should be. Self-compassion leads us back to ourselves. There is a famous children's book, *Little I-Am-Me*. A mythical creature is asked by a fish what sort of animal it is. Until then it hasn't cared about its identity at all. Now it has doubts and sets off to find its roots. It goes on to question many different animals. All of them find something about it that excludes it from being a member of that particular species. It has a horse's tail, but its body is checked, so it can't be a horse. And so on. The fantasy animal gets more and more desperate. Suddenly it realises: 'I am me. I am unique and I don't have to be another animal.'

This is also the essence of self-compassion: you find out who you really are, what you really need, and what you can do without. With this knowledge you can then take better care of yourself.

This also means forgiving yourself when you behave badly, which may be due to a stressful situation, physical or mental health stressors, and/or your hormone imbalance. Don't condemn yourself for your own actions. The situation has gone badly enough. Mindfulness and self-compassion go hand in hand here. Ask yourself, *what just happened, how did it come about, what could go better the next time, and how can I apologise or take responsibility for the situation?* Otherwise, we are back to the question of setting boundaries. Saying no, as we have seen, is also part of practising self-compassion.

Say goodbye to the belief that 'If I just try a bit harder, everything will be fine, and I will be loved and accepted.' This is rubbish. You don't need to follow the maxim 'Bad girls go everywhere', but you should dare to be authentic, be yourself, and listen to your gut. If your gut increasingly becomes cramped or your throat constricts, then you may need to get out of the situation or the relationship.

Don't wait too long to change behaviour that makes you ill — and try to let go of feeling guilty about it. One of the reasons why women are so likely to suffer from anxiety and depression is the endless tossing and turning of thoughts, usually before falling asleep at night. This is probably ingrained through a culture that expects perfection and endless free emotional labour from us. This kind of brooding negatively affects our mental and physical health. Sleep should be regarded as sacred because, as we showed in Chapter 3, cell repair and stress regeneration take place at night.

Self-compassion and learning true self-care are the best tools for stress prevention, and for promoting relaxation and a healthy self-esteem. They help us to find our balance again during the turbulent time of hormonal change.

QUESTIONNAIRE:
HOW MUCH SELF-COMPASSION DO I HAVE?

Consider these questions carefully. How many of them resonate with you? Does answering them truthfully show you ways you might be kinder to yourself?

- Am I my own worst critic?
- Can I forgive myself?
- Can I figuratively give myself a hug to cheer myself up?
- Do I take my own needs seriously?
- Do I see and appreciate my achievements?
- Do I think of myself kindly?
- Do I use kind words when I talk about myself?
- Can I accept praise and compliments?

I AM WORTH IT: HEALTHY SELF-WORTH

Many of us judge ourselves very harshly, and without reason. If we are given a compliment on our appearance, we immediately respond with, 'Do you think so? My face is so puffy today', or 'I missed out on a job recently, things aren't great ...'

This kind of self-criticism is known as *talking yourself down,* a strategy that becomes self-destructive sooner or later. You are what you think or, in other words, if you consider yourself to be an unlovable person for many years, then the chances are you will become an exhausting grump. Women in particular tend to elevate their inner critic into prime position. Some women like to put the focus on their own weaknesses. This is often due to negative self-perception. You play down your strengths — and everybody has considerable strengths.

In our society, envy and fear of exclusion are strong drivers for the need to please everyone. When instead you allow yourself to be praised, you immediately feel odd.

Self-criticism can also be deceptive: it gets in the way of what is actually true and important. If I put myself down, then the other person's reaction can only be ramped up: 'No really, I mean it, you look great today!' And you've probably already counter-complimented them — 'I don't look good, but you do.'

People who have a firmly established value system can go through life with more independence from external influences. A pejorative remark does not leave them feeling downcast or drained of energy. They know what is important in their lives.

SKB: 'In my professional and personal spheres, I know of many people who doubt themselves. Surprisingly, this is even true of those who are successful lawyers, teachers, doctors, and wonderful parents. I can see that self-esteem does not depend on bank balances or on a stable marriage, or anything else besides. You often hear people say: "What did I ever achieve?" A question put to themselves that is meant to be disparaging. My sincere response in lectures and to my friends is: "Be kinder to yourself. Look back and list everything that you've done, even the normal things you do every day, and things you take for granted. Be proud of yourself and don't doubt yourself so much." People often look at me in bewilderment. The idea of being gracious to yourself includes mercy and compassion. For many, this idea, in relation to themselves, is something that has never occurred to them before. "Interesting," is the usual reply. Yes, very interesting and very true!'

Many women naturally possess excellent social skills: creativity, empathy, and sensitivity, all sorts of important qualities that hold us together as a society and which should be encouraged. Unfortunately, for many women who live alone following a separation or a divorce, their self-esteem sinks rapidly. Without a partner by their side, some women only feel half as valued as a woman and therefore as a human being. Their self-worth is based on a fragile foundation. If their partner breaks away, the woman breaks too because she's always defined herself through her partnership or her family. This is called external identification. This is sad because every single person is without a doubt a valuable person with a million interesting qualities that continue to exist regardless of whether they are partnered or not.

The principle of external identification is true of other parts of life, too. Often the need for recognition and confirmation is at the forefront. If someone feels this appreciation is not forthcoming because they have lost their job, for example, then this not only leads to justified frustration and worry, but often also fundamentally damages their self-esteem. In addition to unemployment, a personal crisis can result.

Even if we know that it's easier said than done, it is extremely important for your self-esteem that you build a sense of self-worth that's not dependent on external validation. We should do the things we do for ourselves with complete conviction, regardless of whether there is someone standing next to us applauding or not. When we have achieved something, we should be happy about it and enjoy our success. The external recognition is then the icing on the cake, but not the cake itself.

We could all use more lightness, humour, praise, and appreciation. However, many women find it hard to accept praise. How do you deal with praise? Was a lot of praise given in your family home or was there just criticism? Do you receive recognition from the people who are close to you? Are you praised by others and, if not, do you praise yourself (*I managed to do that? I am really proud of myself!*) No? Then it's high time you did!

WHERE TO GO WITH YOUR ANGER?

We'd like to address another topic that menopausal women keep asking us about: anger. Anger can gnaw at our self-esteem. Many women in their forties say: 'I am sooo angry'. If you ask them why, there are many different answers: life, men, parents-in-law, bosses, the weather, a bad movie, missed opportunities, growing old, or putting on weight. But above all it's anger about having spent so many years being used by those around them so self-evidently and then being left with what feels like nothing afterwards. *Why did I do all that, and why didn't anyone else help? Why didn't I resist or refuse? Why was I the unwise one? Why am I not secure, or independent, or financially stable?*

Dealing with your own anger can be very healing, including in the medical sense. Spiritually, it leads us back to ourselves.

Anger has two main causes: either you feel personally belittled, attacked, or disrespectfully treated, or perhaps your own expectations were disappointed, or the other person reacted differently from how you imagined they would. In the first case, we would say it was intentional: 'Eva knew full well that she was going to hurt me with this. Peter deliberately insulted me. Lula knows how to wind me up'. The weaker your self-esteem, the more quickly and easily you'll feel hurt and put out by another person or a situation (bad weather, the late train, the traffic jam). But maybe the other person was just having a bad day, or was inattentive or thoughtless because they were thinking about what they might give their partner for their birthday. Or maybe they were tense because of an upcoming dental appointment.

Ask yourself why your environment and the people around you infuriate you so much and whether or not they were actually acting in a malicious, bullying way. Probably not. Neither do the weather, the train delay or the traffic jam on the motorway have anything to do with you. The world is always spinning, things happen, and you are rarely the centre of attention. Attention or sympathy from others often only comes in the moments of greatest success and defeat. Others briefly raise their heads, only to then return to their own life again. 'Did something happen?'

However, when your own expectations are disappointed by another person time and again, and this makes you angry, then you should give your behaviour an honest examination. Is the expectation in someone or something realistic, fair, and justified? Is it even possible to meet your demand or fulfil your request in the given time? The answers to these honest questions may not be favourable to you. Unfortunately, this is not unusual.

Is the anger that you feel towards others perhaps anger with yourself? It's worth taking a closer look at the anger trap. Everyone gets angry sometimes — you don't need to be embarrassed about it, and you shouldn't suppress anger. Let it all out. Being angry can release energy in order to continue with difficult conversations or to free yourself from unbearable situations and build a new life. In this sense, anger can be quite healing and highlight your own needs.

But forgive yourself for your anger and try to let it go if it is self-destructive (and if necessary, apologise when you have been unreasonably angry with someone). This is the only way to avoid becoming a victim of your own negative feelings, which are feelings of powerlessness and loss of control. A useful trick to help you get out of the 'I-am-so-furious-because-I'm-disappointed-about-the-world' attitude is to change the words and, best of all, address it directly: 'It would be nice if you could help me tomorrow with the shopping.' This is better than having disappointed, angry thoughts about your partner because once again they didn't offer to help without needing any prompting ('the jerk, typical, they should have known!').

'I wish ...' is also very effective.

In cases of frequent or permanent feelings of anger, it makes sense to try to breathe away the anger or internally 'smile' it away. If you learn to practise this, the brain learns to vent the anger.

There are, of course, also very serious traumatic reasons for anger, such as abuse or grief. In these cases, anger is the expression of your own powerlessness. You could benefit from the support of a good counsellor. In such cases we would strongly recommend you seek psychological help.

Dealing with anger also means being able to forgive. It is important for your own peace of mind to be able to forgive those who you feel have hurt you, such as an ex-partner, for example. Naturally there are limits here, too. A criminal who has caused serious personal suffering to you, your family or other people does not need to be forgiven. If you do, however, manage to do this, then this is evidence of (super) human greatness. And just because you forgive someone, it doesn't mean you ever need to engage with them again or accept their poor behaviour. You can be forgiving and maintain firm boundaries at the same time.

In the other cases, you will be able to live with your anger and yourself better if you recognise that you did your best in the situation at the time. It's always easy to blame yourself in retrospect. But try to remind yourself that in the past you had less knowledge and wisdom, which was why your decisions at the time were the only ones possible and therefore also the best you could do.

IT'S MY TURN NOW

We have returned to this idea throughout the book because it is typically a female issue and it keeps coming up. Women tend to care about everything and everyone, but not about themselves. After several decades of worrying and caring, many women feel exhausted and frustrated. But especially in mid life, being aware of your own needs, without any exaggeration, is essential for survival. If hormonal changes have left you feeling weak and exhausted or even ill, then it is high time to take care of yourself. We would like to encourage you to do so without feeling guilty.

What throws you off track and into chaos, what gets on your nerves, and what saps your strength? The answers to these questions lead to the crux of the matter: what gives you strength?

Now is the time to take stock. Perfectionism to the point of exhaustion no longer makes sense, and neither do hundreds of hours of overtime or leisure activities that you don't actually enjoy. Hours of relationship discussions without any noticeable progress will just lead to you and your partner going around in circles. So, consider going to couples therapy, or give yourself or your partner some space. Maybe you will rediscover why you love each other, and maybe you can start afresh with this love. If not, so be it. The same goes for friendships.

Our tip: For one week, write down everything that you do for others. Don't evaluate it, just write it down. Ideally take a big piece of paper and write down everything — literally everything. All the activities related to your work and personal life: helping out a colleague who needs to leave early, watering your neighbour's plants while they are on holiday, speaking to a family member on the phone, ironing your children's clothes. Then, with a thicker red marker pen, cross out everything that cost you your strength. Carry that list around with you and keep checking it. No doubt several of these items will be missing from the new list you make the following week!

Important decisions are usually not made on a whim, but instead we make them when we can't take anymore or when we are motivated by success. It's like choosing to eat healthier food. Either you get fed up with feeling lethargic and unhealthy, or you've already felt the benefit of a cleaner diet and are motivated to continue. If you have made a decision, then resources are suddenly freed up to support you.

SEB: 'Many women feel trapped on a treadmill between work, family and social obligations. I have never encountered a patient who has not been able to change her life. It was

always possible to at least change the approach or some
of the important aspects. I have met women who had to
get through extremely difficult life situations requiring
huge effort. Surprisingly, none of these women was broken
by these challenges. On the contrary: approaching and
overcoming the situation showed the women how strong
they were. Their personal path suddenly became a lot clearer,
more satisfying and — despite what initially looked like
difficult circumstances — often happier too.'

In the past, menopause was known as the 'dangerous age' (for
husbands and partners, mind you!). Women do indeed experience
creative momentum and they set off on new challenges. Many
surpass their expectations of themselves. This is one of the reasons
why so many women in mid life go on training courses to get a new
qualification, or go for an exciting career change. Those around
them are often amazed. We don't want to drive up the divorce rate
here — on the contrary. It would just be nice if a woman's personal
development could include their partner and would lead to inspir-
ing conversations and new joint ventures.

You don't need to make a clean sweep and spectacularly tear
down everything that you've built up over decades. A (re)filled life
is often just a life with a new or stronger consciousness. We all have
a deep knowledge about what is important to us and *why* we aspire
to do something. This knowledge has not been lost but has just been
buried under the weight of external obligations.

HOW CAN YOU TAKE GOOD CARE OF YOURSELF?

Letting go and delegating are important measures. Self-care goes
beyond that because it also includes fulfilment and happiness.

Middle age offers an incredible opportunity to enter into a deep
dialogue with yourself, to listen to your own wishes, and realise
your ideas. This includes a pinch of selfishness, not at the cost of

others, but also for your own benefit. Small changes create big steps. Which obligations do you meet simply out of habit and feel miserable about? What tires you out? What makes you angry? What do you wish for, what do you need, what wishes can you fulfil with the means that you have? What do you dream about, what can you now dare to do?

Hungarian psychologist Mihály Csíkszentmihályi coined the term *flow* as experiencing 'a state in which people are so involved in an activity that nothing else seems to matter; the experience is so enjoyable that people will continue to do it even at great cost, for the sheer sake of doing it'.

What puts you in flow? How do you find your personal happiness? Bhutan is the only country in the world with gross national happiness as a state goal. There is no general happiness formula that applies to everyone, but it is undisputed that humans who can actively shape their own lives are happier than those who feel a permanent sense of alienation. Those who insist that happiness must come to them from something external, whether that is through a partner, an inheritance to which they think they are entitled, or other things that are 'owed', are usually headed straight for misfortune. The conviction that others are responsible for your happiness inevitably leads to disappointment and frustration. Single people who dream of the happiness of a fulfilling relationship have to play their part too. It's not enough to find your Prince or Princess Charming.

Fortunately, in this country, people are becoming less materialistic. Status symbols are losing their exaggerated value. Generation Z has a different idea of healthy work–life–balance, including things like car sharing, short-term housing, and flexible work arrangements.

By nature, humans are social beings and therefore happier when embedded in a circle of family and friends, rather than alone. Being able to accept yourself with all your strengths and weaknesses — that is an important pillar. And another is: enjoying the good things in life and reconciling yourself with the negative things.

Everyone has to find their own way through the jungle of life. Many people constantly live in a state of *if–then*. If I become a successful lawyer, then I'll be happy; if I finally get my dream house, then I'll be content, and so on. The successful Swiss author Rolf Dobelli holds the view that plans hardly ever work out. They have to be constantly corrected, renewed, and adapted. Those who make their happiness conditional, and then freeze in a state of inflexibility when these conditions don't come to pass, are more likely to be dissatisfied and sad than happy and fulfilled.

Scientific studies have shown that it doesn't take much to be happy. Experiences lead to more sustainable happiness than possessions, status, admiration, or external recognition. Inner contemplation and meditation pave the way for a happy life; so do small things, such as an attentive word from your partner, a warm hug, a flower to place on the table, an evening with friends, and laughing together. Peace with your fellow humans, the feeling of being in harmony with your own values, and being able to live with nature are also part of this.

Close your eyes and think of a very happy moment in your life: what is still here, and what is now absent? What is worthwhile keeping fit, or getting healthy and fit, for? What is really important to you?

If you follow your heart in this way, then you will find a feeling of harmony. Harmony begins with ourselves and spreads from there to our fellow human beings and our surroundings.

Let's recap: self-care means taking your own needs seriously, creating space and safe havens, allowing yourself to be happy, getting into the flow, and dreaming — of happiness, of love, of lightness, of inner freedom, of setting off and arriving.

We wish you much joy on your very own personal journey!

Acknowledgements

We would like to thank all the women whose stories, experiences, and challenges have inspired us to write this book. The openness and trust with which they told us about their very personal experiences moved us and kept us going, especially during those times when everyday madness threatened to collide with our writing flow.

We thank our mentors, colleagues, and supporters. We would particularly like to thank our agent, Dr Hanna Leitgeb, who put in a huge amount of effort for us.

We would like to thank the wonderful team at Lübbe, who captured our hearts and with whom we experienced wonderful moments this year. We would particularly like to thank our editor, Franziska Beyer, for her great commitment, her passion for the subject, and her creativity. She has made it possible for us to implement all the ideas we had for the book.

During the intensive writing phase in our homes in Berlin, we were driven by the curiosity and huge interest from our friends, siblings, parents, and the community. Thank you to Sabine and Jürgen for the circus caravan-writing room in the Swedish garden. SEB: Thank you, Robert, for your support.

Our final thanks go to the next generation — our children, Lilly,

Carlotta, David, and Luca, who as the Fridays-for-Future generation are also interested in this subject.

Sources

CHAPTER 1 INTRODUCTION

Burger, H.G. et al.: Hormonal changes in the menopause transition. *Recent Progress in Hormone Research* 2002; 57: 257–275

Mishra, G.D. et al.: Early menarche, nulliparity and the risk for premature and early natural menopause. *Human Reproduction* 2017; 32 (3): 679–686

Woods, N.F. et al.: Cortisol levels during the menopausal transition and early postmenopause: observations from the Seattle Midlife Women's Health Study. *Menopause* 2009; 16 (4): 708–718

CHAPTER 2 THE HORMONE CAROUSEL

Avis, N.E. et al.: Duration of menopausal vasomotor symptoms over the menopause transition. *JAMA Internal Medicine* 2015; 175 (4): 531–539

Christensen, K. et al.: Perceived age as clinically useful biomarker of ageing: cohort study. *British Medical Journal* 2009; 339: b5262

Lindheim, L. et al.: Alterations in gut microbiome composition and barrier function are associated with reproductive and metabolic defects in women with polycystic ovary syndrome (PCOS): a pilot study. *PLoS One* 2017; 12 (1): e0168390

Mark Park, Y. et al.: Association of exposure to artificial light at night while sleeping with risk of obesity in women. *JAMA Internal Medicine* 2019;179 (8): 1061–1071

Rapkin, A.J. et al.: Pathophysiology of premenstrual syndrome and premenstrual dysphoric disorder. *Menopause International* 2012; 18 (2): 52–59

CHAPTER 3 BALANCING OUR HORMONES — THIS IS HOW IT WORKS

Asi, N. et al.: Progesterone vs. synthetic progestins and the risk of breast cancer: a systematic review and meta-analysis. *Systematic Reviews* 2016; 5 (1): 121

Bakken, K. et al.: Menopausal hormone therapy and breast cancer risk: impact of different treatments. The European Prospective Investigation into Cancer and Nutrition. *International Journal of Cancer* 2011; 128 (1): 144–156

Beral, V. et al.: Breast cancer and hormone-replacement therapy in the Million Women Study. *The Lancet* 2003; 362 (9382): 419–427

Björnsdottir, S. et al.: Risk of hip fracture in Addison's disease: a population-based cohort study. *Journal of Internal Medicine* 2011; 270 (2): 187–195

Björntorp, P. et al.: Obesity and cortisol. *Nutrition* 2000; 16 (10): 924–936

Boursi, B. et al.: Thyroid dysfunction, thyroid hormone replacement, and colorectal cancer risk. *Journal of the National Cancer Institute* 2015; 107 (6): djv084

Brinkman, M.T. et al.: Consumption of animal products, their nutrient components and postmenopausal circulating steroid hormone concentrations. *European Journal of Clinical Nutrition* 2010; 64 (2): 176–183

Brunt, V.E. et al.: Suppression of the gut microbiome ameliorates age-related arterial dysfunction and oxidative stress in mice. *Journal of Physiology* 2019; 597 (9): 2361–2378

Canonico, M. et al.: Postmenopausal hormone therapy and risk of stroke: impact of the route of estrogen administration and type of progestogen. *Stroke* 2016; 47 (7): 1734-1741

Caufriez, A, et al.: Progesterone prevents sleep disturbances and modulates GH, TSH, and melatonin secretion in postmenopausal women. *Journal of Clinical Endocrinology and Metabolism* 2011; 96 (4): 614-623

Chlebowski, R. et al.: Breast cancer after use of estrogen plus progestin in postmenopausal women. *The New England Journal of Medicine* 2009; 360 (6): 573-587

Collaborative Group on Hormonal Factors in Breast Cancer: Type and timing of menopausal hormone therapy and breast cancer risk: individual participant meta-analysis of the worldwide epidemiological evidence. *The Lancet* 2019; 394 (8): 1159-1168

Cordina-Duverger, E. et al.: Risk of breast cancer by type of menopausal hormone therapy: a case-control study among post-menopausal women in France. *PLoS One* 2013; 8 (11): E78016

Dalessandri, K.M. et al.: Pilot study: effect of 3,3'-diindolylmethane supplements on urinary hormone metabolites in postmenopausal women with a history of early-stage breast cancer. *Nutrition and Cancer* 2004; 50 (2): 161-167

De Lignières, B. et al.: Combined hormone replacement therapy and risk of breast cancer in a French cohort study of 3175 women. *Climacteric* 2002; 5 (4): 332-340

Del Priore, G. et al.: Oral diindolylmethane (DIM): pilot evaluation of a nonsurgical treatment for cervical dysplasia. *Gynecologic Oncology* 2010; 116 (3): 464-467

Epel, E.S. et al.: Accelerated telomere shortening in response to life stress. *Proceedings of the National Academy of Sciences of the United States of America* 2004; 101 (49): 17312-17315

Espinoza, T.R. et al.: The role of progesterone in traumatic brain injury. *Journal of Head Trauma Rehabilitation* 2011; 26 (6): 497-499

Farhat, G.N. et al.: Sex hormone levels and risks of estrogen receptor-negative and estrogen receptor-positive breast cancers. *Journal of the National Cancer Institute* 2011; 103 (7) 201: 562–570

Fasano, A.: Leaky gut and autoimmune diseases. *Clinical Reviews in Allergy & Immunology* 2012; 42 (1): 71–80

Fournier, A. et al.: Risks of endometrial cancer associated with different hormone replacement therapies in the E3N cohort, 1992–2008. *American Journal of Epidemiology*. 2014; 180 (5): 508–517

Fournier, A. et al.: Unequal risks for breast cancer associated with different hormone replacement therapies: results from the E3N cohort study. *Breast Cancer and Research Treatment* 2008; 107(1): 103–111

Gemeinsame Stellungnahme der Deutschen Gesellschaft für Gynäkologische Endokrinologie und Fortpflanzungsmedizin (DGGEF) und des Berufsverbands der Frauenärzte (BVF) e.V.: Management von Endometriumhyperplasien. *Journal für Reproduktionsmedizin und Endokrinologie* 2014; 11 (4): 170–185

Harach, T. et al.: Reduction of Abeta amyloid pathology in APPPS1 transgenic mice in the absence of gut microbiota. *Scientific Reports* 2017; 7: Artikel nr. 41802

Hodis, H.N. et al.: A 'window of opportunity': the reduction of coronary heart disease and total mortality with menopausal therapies is age- and time-dependent. *Brain Research* 2011; 1379: 244–252

Hughes, J.W. et al.: Depression and anxiety symptoms are related to increased 24-hour urinary norepinephrine excretion among healthy middle-aged women. *Journal of Psychosomatic Research* 2004; 57 (4): 353–358

Huiying, Y. et al.: Regulated inflammation and lipid metabolism in colon mRNA expressions of obese germfree mice responding to enterobacter cloacae B29 combined with the high fat diet. *Frontiers in Microbiology* 2016; 7: 1786

Imtiaz, B.: Risk of Alzheimer's disease among users of postmenopausal hormone therapy: A nationwide case-control study. *Maturitas* 2017; 98: 7–13

Kaur, J. et al.: Association of vitamin D status with chronic disease risk factors and cognitive dysfunction in 50–70 year old adults. *Nutrients* 2019; 11 (1): E 141

Kleine-Gunk, B.: Anti-Aging-Medizin — Hoffnung oder Humbug? *Deutsches Ärzteblatt* 2007; 104 (28–29): 2054–2060

Leitlinienprogramm, Deutsche Gesellschaft für Gynäkologie und Geburtshilfe (DGGG): Peri- und Postmenopause — Diagnostik und Interventionen, *AWMF* online 2018

L'hermite, M. et al.: Could transdermal estradiol + progesterone be a safer postmenopausal HRT? A review. *Maturitas* 2008; 60 (3–4): 185–201

Li, C.I. et al.: Alcohol consumption and risk of postmenopausal breast cancer by subtype: the Women's Health Initiative observational study. *Journal of the National Cancer Institute* 2010; 102 (18): 1422–1431

Liu, B.: Is transdermal menopausal hormone therapy a safer option than oral therapy? *Canadian Medical Association Journal* 2013; 185 (7): 549–550

Løkkegaard, E. et al.: Hormone therapy and risk of myocardial infarction: a national register study. *European Heart Journal* 2008; 29 (21): 2660–2668

Løkkegaard, E. et al.: Risk of stroke with various types of menopausal hormone therapies: a national cohort study. *Stroke* 2017; 48 (8): 2266–2269

Manson, J.E.: Menopausal hormone therapy and health outcomes during the intervention and extended poststopping phases of the Women's Health Initiative randomized trials. *JAMA* 2013; 310 (13): 1353–1368

Manson, J.E. et al.: Menopausal hormone therapy and long-term all-cause and cause-specific mortality: the Women's Health Initiative randomized trials. *JAMA* 2017; 318 (10): 927–938

Manson, J.E. et al.: Menopause management — getting clinical care back on track. *The New England Journal of Medicine* 2016; 374(9): 803–806

Marculescu, R. et al.: Vitamin D deficiency tied to risk for diabetes death. *Präsentation der Daten auf dem European Association for the Study of Diabetes Annual Meeting*, Barcelona 2019

Mason, C. et al.: Vitamin D3 supplementation during weight loss: a double-blind randomized controlled trial. *American Journal of Clinical Nutrition* 2014; 99 (5): 1015-1025

Meloun, M. et al.: Minimizing the effects of multicollinearity in the polynomial regression of age relationships and sex differences in serum levels of pregnenolone sulfate in healthy subjects. *Clinical Chemistry and Laboratory Medicine* 2009; 47 (4): 464-470

Meybohm, P. et al.: Effekt von hochdosiertem Vitamin D3 auf die 28-Tage Mortalität bei erwachsenen kritisch kranken Patienten mit schwerem Vitamin D Mangel: eine multizentrische, Placebo-kontrollierte, doppelblinde Phase III Studie. Uniklinik Frankfurt, Klinik für Anästhesiologie, Intensivmedizin und Schmerztherapie, Laufende Studie 2019-2024 Miller H: Response to The bioidentical hormone debate: are bioidentical hormones (estradiol, estriol, and progesterone) safer or more efficacious than commonly used synthetic versions in hormone replacement therapy?". *Postgraduate Medicine* 2009; 121(4): 172

Mishra, G.D. et al.: Hysterectomy trends in Australia, 2000-2001 to 2013-2014: joinpoint regression analysis. *Acta Obstet Gynecol Scand* 2017; 96:1170-1179.

Mueck, A.O.: Hormonsubstitution: WHI-Autoren mahnen: Millionen von Frauen müssen unnötig leiden! *Frauenarzt* 2016; 57 (5): 2-3

Murkes, D. et al.: Effects of percutaneous estradiol-oral progesterone versus oral conjugated equine estrogens-medroxyprogesterone acetate on breast cell proliferation and bcl-2 protein in healthy women. *Fertility and Sterility* 2011; 95(3): 1188-1191

Murkes, D.: Percutaneous estradiol/oral micronized progesterone has less-adverse effects and different gene regulations than oral conjugated equine estrogens/ medroxyprogesterone acetate in the breasts of healthy women in vivo. *Gynecological Endocrinology* 2012; 28 (2): 12-15

Müssig, K. et al.: Thyroid peroxidase antibody positivity is associated with symptomatic distress in patients with Hashimoto's thyroiditis. *Brain, Behavior, and Immunity* 2012; 26 (4): 559-563

Nadkarni S et al.: Activation of the Annexin A1 pathway underlies the protective effects exerted by estrogen in polymorphonuclear leukocytes. *Arteriosclerosis, Thrombosis, and Vascular Biology* 2011; 31 (8): 2749-2759

Nelson, H.D. et al.: Nonhormonal therapies for menopausal hot flashes: systematic review and meta-analysis. *JAMA* 2006; 295 (17): 2057-2071

Olié, V.: Risk of venous thrombosis with oral versus transdermal estrogen therapy among postmenopausal women. *Current Opinion in Hematology* 2010; 17 (5): 457-463

Ortmann, O.: HRT und Krebsrisiko: Was muss ich bei der Vorsorge berücksichtigen. 62. Kongress DGGG 2018, Berlin, Pressetext

Pace-Schott, E.F. et al.: Age-related changes in the cognitive function of sleep. *Progress Brain Research* 2011; 191: 75-89

Prentice, R.L. et al.: Benefits and risks of postmenopausal hormone therapy when it is initiated soon after menopause. *American Journal of Epidemiology* 2009; 170 (1): 12-23

Renoux, C. et al.: Transdermal and oral hormone replacement therapy and the risk of stroke: a nested case-control study. *British Medical Journal* 2010; 340: C2519

Römmler, A. et al.: Progesteron: Genitale und extragenitale Wirkungen. *Zeitschrift für Orthomolekulare Medizin* 2009; 7 (3): 9-13

Rossouw, J.E. et al.: Risks and benefits of estrogen plus progestin in healthy postmenopausal women: principal results from the Women's Health Initiative randomized controlled trial. *JAMA* 2001; 288 (3): 321-333

Scarabin, P.Y.: Progestogens and venous thromboembolism in menopausal women: an updated oral versus transdermal estrogen meta-analysis. *Climacteric* 2018; 21 (4) 341-351

Schaudig, K. et al.: Individualisierte Hormontherapie in Peri- und Postmenopause. *Gynäkologische Endokrinologie* 2016; 14: 31-43 Stute, P. et al.: The impact of micronized progesterone on the endometrium: a systematic review. *Climacteric* 2016; 19 (4): 316-328

Schlehe, J.S. et al.: Das Mikrobiom: Einfluss auf Adipositas und Diabetes. *Deutsches Ärzteblatt* 2016; 113 (17): 27

Shao, H. et al.: Hormone therapy and Alzheimer disease dementia: new findings from the Cache County Study. *Neurology* 2012; 79 (18): 1846-1852

Simon, J.A.: What if the Women's Health Initiative had used transdermal estradiol and oral progesterone instead? *Menopause* 2014; 21 (7): 769-783

Sisto, M. et al.: Proposing a relationship between Mycobacterium avium subspecies paratuberculosis infection and Hashimoto's thyroiditis. *Scandinavian Journal of Infectious Diseases* 2010; 42 (10): 787-790

Sturdee, D.W. et al.: Recommendations for the management to post-menopausal vaginal atrophy. *Climacteric* 2010; 13 (6): 509-522

Stute, P. et al.: The impact of micronized progesterone on breast cancer risk: a systematoc review. *Climacteric* 2018; 21 (2) 111-122

Theis, V.C.: VEGF und Progesteron. Ruhr-Universität Bochum, Abteilung Cytologie, *AG Strukturelle Plastizität*, 2017

Thurston, R.C. et al.: Adiposity and reporting of vasomotor symptoms among midlife women: the study of women's health across the nation. *American Journal of Epidemiology* 2008; 167(1): 78-85

Trummer. C. et al.: Effects of vitamin D supplementation on metabolic and endocrine parameters in PCOS: a randomized-controlled trial. *European Journal of Nutrition* 2019; 58 (5): 2019-2028

Wallwiener M: Medikamentöse konservative Therapie des Uterus myomatosus. *Der Gynäkologe* 2019; 4

Wang, H. et al.: Bifidobacterium longum 1714™ strain modulates brain activity of healthy volunteers during social stress. *American Journal of Gastroenterology* 2019; 114 (7): 1152-1162

Wenderlein, J.M.: Hormonelle Darmkrebsprävention. *Deutsches Ärzteblatt International* 2014; 114: 426-427

Wenderlein, J.M.: Östrogentherapie nicht vergessen. *Deutsches Ärzteblatt International* 2012; 109 (42): 714

Women's Health Initiative Steering Committee: Effects of conjugated equine estrogen in postmenopausal women with hysterectomy: The Women's Health Initiative randomized controlled trial. *JAMA* 2004; 291(14): 1701-1712

Wren, B.G. et al.: Transdermal progesterone and its effect on vasomotor symptoms, blood lipid levels, bone metabolic markers, moods, and quality of life for postmenopausal women. *Menopause* 2003; 10 (1): 13–18

Zaletel, K. et al.: Hashimoto's Thyroiditis: from genes to the disease. *Current Genomics* 2011; 12 (8): 576–588

Zamani, M. et al.: Therapeutic effect of Vitex agnus castus in patients with premenstrual syndrome. *Acta Medica Iranica* 2012; 50 (2): 101–106

Zylka-Menhorn, V.: Aus der Forschung: Metformin verändert die Darmflora. *Deutsches Ärzteblatt* 2016; 113 (43): 32

CHAPTER 4 EXTERNAL HORMONE MANIPULATION

Bellas, J. et al.: Ingestion of microplastics by demersal fish from the Spanish Atlantic and Mediterranean coasts. *Marine Pollution Bulletin* 2016; 109: 55–60

Carwile, J.L.: Canned soup consumption and urinary bisphenol A: a randomized crossover trial. *Journal of the American Medical Association.* 2011, 306 (20): 2218–2220

Chen, Q. et al.: Sperm tsRNAs contribute to intergenerational inheritance of an acquired metabolic disorder. *Science.* 2016; 351 (6271): 397–400

De Agüero, M.G.: The maternal microbiota drives early postnatal innate immune development. *Science* 2016; 351(6279): 1296–1302

Deutsche Gesellschaft für Endokrinologie (DGE): Lifestyle und Umwelteinflüsse verursachen Volkskrankheiten: Experten diskutieren Rolle chronischer Entzündungsreaktionen. 2018; 61. Kongress für Endokrinologie der DGE

Europäische Kommission: Für einen umfassenden Rahmen der Europäischen Union für endokrine Disruptoren. COM 2018; 734 final Report United Nations Environment Programme: Plastic in cosmetics: are we polluting the environment through our personal care: plastic ingredients that contribute to marine microplastic litter. *UNEP*; letzte Version 2017

Franklin, T.: Epigenetic transmission of the impact of early stress across generations. *Biological Psychiatry* 2010; 68 (5): 408–415

Gallo, M.V. et al.: Endocrine disrupting chemicals and ovulation: Is there a relationship? *Environmental Research* 2016; 151: 410–418

Gore, A.C.: Neuroendocrine targets of endocrine disruptors. *Hormones* 2010; 9 (1): 16–27

Jedeon, K. et al.: Systemic enamel pathologies may be due to anti-androgenic effects of some endocrine disruptors. *Endocrine Abstracts* 2016; 41: OC10.1

Kandaraki, E.: Endocrine disruptors and polycystic ovary syndrome (PCOS): elevated serum levels of bisphenol A in women with PCOS. *Journal of Clinical Endocrinology & Metabolism* 2011; 96 (3): E480–E484

Klöting, N .et al.: Di-(2-Ethylhexyl)-Phthalate (DEHP) causes impaired adipocyte function and alters serum metabolites. *PLoS One.* 2015; 10 (12): e0143190.

La Merrill, M.A. et al.: The economic legacy of endocrine-disrupting chemicals. *The Lancet Diabetes & Endocrinology* 2016; 4 (12): 961–962

Lang, I.A. et al.: »Association of urinary bisphenol A concentration with medical disorders and laboratory abnormalities in adults.« *JAMA* 2008; 300 (11): 1303–1310

Lönnstedt, O.M. et al.: Environmentally relevant concentrations of microplastic particles influence larval fish ecology. *Science* 2016; 352 (6290): 1213–1216

Manikkam, M.: Plastics derived endocrine disruptors (BPA, DEHP and DBP) induce epigenetic transgenerational inheritance of obesity, reproductive disease and sperm epimutations. *PLoS One* 2013; 8 (1): e55387

Michaëlsson, K.: Milk intake and risk of mortality and fractures in women and men: cohort studies. *British Medical Journal* 2014; 349: g6015

Neel, B.A. et al.: »The paradox of progress: environmental disruption of metabolism and the diabetes epidemic.« *Diabetes* 2011; 60 (7): 1838–1848

Okbay A et al.: Genetic variants associated with subjective well-being, depressive symptoms, and neuroticism identified through genome-wide analyses. *Nature Genetics* 2016; 48: 624–633

Rasic-Milutinovic, Z. et al.: Potential influence of selenium, copper, zinc and cadmium on L-Thyroxine substitution in patients with Hashimoto Thyroiditis and hypothyroidism. *Experimental and Clinical Endocrinology & Diabetes* 2017; 125 (02): 79–85

Ringrose, L.: Distinct contributions of histone H3 lysine 9 and 27 methylation to locus-specific stability of polycomb complexes. *Molecular Cell*, 2004; 16 (4): 641–653

Schwabl, P. et al.: Detection of various microplastics in human stool: a prospective case series. *Annals of Internal Medicine* 2019; 9 453–57

Siklenka, K. et al.: Disruption of histone methylation in developing sperm impairs offspring health transgenerationally. *Science*. 2015; 350 (6261): aab2006

Umweltbewusstseinsstudie 2018 vom Bundesministerium für Umwelt, Naturschutz und nukleare Sicherheit: Bevölkerung erwartet mehr Umwelt- und Klimaschutz von allen Akteuren. *Veröffentlicht*: 5/2019

Wang, G. et al.: Association between maternal prepregnancy body mass index and plasma folate concentrations with child metabolic health. *JAMA Pediatrics* 2016; 170 (8): e160845

Wieczorek, A.M.: Frequency of microplastics in mesopelagic fishes from the Northwest Atlantic. *Frontiers in Marine Science* 2018, Originalartikel

CHAPTER 5 SELF-CARE

Adler-Neal, A.L. et al.: The role of heart rate variability in mindfulness-based pain relief. *Journal of Pain* 2019; pii: S1526–5900 (19): 30773–4

Anheyer D et al.: Mindfulness-based stress reduction for treating low back pain: a systematic review and meta-analysis. *Annals of Internal Medicine* 2017; 166 (11): 799–807

Banasik, J. et al.: Effect of Iyengar yoga practice on fatigue and diurnal salivary cortisol concentration in breast cancer survivors. *Journal of the American Academy of Nurse Practitioners* 2011; 23 (3): 135–142

Bateson, M.: Cumulative stress in research animals: Telomere attrition as a biomarker in a welfare context? *Bioessays* 2016; 38 (2): 201–212

Benias, P.C. et al.: Structure and distribution of an unrecognized interstitium in human tissues. *Nature, Scientific Reports* 2018; volume 8; Article number 4947

Black, D.S. et al.: Mindfulness meditation and the immune system: a systematic review of randomized controlled trials. *Annals of the New York Academy of Sciences* 2016; 1373 (1): 13–24

Chen, W.Y. et al.: Moderate alcohol consumption during adult life, drinking patterns, and breast cancer risk. *JAMA.* 2011; 306 (17): 1884–1890

Cramer, H. et al.: Yoga bei arterieller Hypertonie. *Deutsches Ärzteblatt International* 2018; 115: 833–839

Cramer, H. et al.: Yoga for improving health-related quality of life, mental health and cancer-related symptoms in women diagnosed with breast cancer. *Cochrane Database Systematic Reviews* 2017; 1: CD010802

Daubenmier, J. et al.: Mindfulness intervention for stress eating to reduce cortisol and abdominal fat among overweight and obese women: an exploratory randomized controlled study. *Journal of Obesity*, 2011, Artikel ID: 651936

Fox, K.C. et al.: Functional neuroanatomy of meditation: A review and meta-analysis of 78 functional neuroimaging investigations. *Neuroscience & Biobehavioral Reviews* 2016; 65 (6): 208–228

Goldstein, P. et al.: The role of touch in regulating inter-partner physiological coupling during empathy for pain. *Nature, Scientific Reports* 2017; volume 7; Article number 3252

Gopal, A. et al.: Effect of integrated yoga practices on immune responses in examination stress — A preliminary study. *International Journal of Yoga* 2011; 4(1): 26–32

Hall A et al.: Effectiveness of tai chi for chronic musculoskeletal pain conditions: updated systematic review and meta-analysis. *Physical Therapy* 2017; 97 (2): 227–238

Heikkila, K. et al.: Long working hours and cancer risk: a multi-cohort study. *British Journal of Cancer* 2016; 114 (7): 813–818

Jacobs, T.L. et al.: Intensive meditation training, immune cell telomerase activity, and psychological mediators. *Psychoneuroendocrinology* 2011; 36 (5): 664–681

Kim, T.W. et al.: The impact of sleep and circadian disturbance on hormones and metabolism. *International Journal of Endocrinology* 2015, Article ID 591729

Kini, P. et al.: The effects of gratitude expression on neural activity. *Neuroimage.* 2016; 128: 1–10

Kivimäki, M. et al.: Long working hours and risk of coronary heart disease and stroke: a systematic review and meta-analysis of published and unpublished data for 603,838 individuals. *The Lancet* 2015; 386 (31): 1739–1746

Korponay, C.: The effect of mindfulness meditation on impulsivity and its neurobiological correlates in healthy adults. *Nature Scientific Reports* 2019; 9: Article number: 11963

Krishna, B.H. et al.: Association of leukocyte telomere length with oxidative stress in yoga practitioners. *Journal of Clinical and Diagnostic Research* 2015; 9 (3): CC01–3

Kwa, M. et al.: The intestinal microbiome and estrogen receptor-positive female breast cancer. *Journal of the National Cancer Institute* 2016; 108 (8)

Le Nguyen, K.D.: Loving-kindness meditation slows biological aging in novices: evidence from a 12-week randomized controlled trial. *Psychoneuroendocrinology* 2019; 108: 20–27

Leger, D. et al.: The role of sleep in the regulation of body weight. *Molecular and Cellular Endocrinology* 2015; 418 (2): 101–107

Lim ,D. et al.: Suffering and compassion: The links among adverse life experiences, empathy, compassion, and prosocial behavior. *Emotion* 2016; 16 (2): 175–182

Linde, K. et al.: Acupuncture for the prevention of episodic migraine. *Cochrane Database Systematic Reviews* 2016; 28 (6): CD001218

Oliveira, B.S. et al.: Systematic review of the association between chronic social stress and telomere length: A life course perspective. *Aging Research Reviews* 26 (3) 2016: 37–52

Puhlmann, L.M. et al.: Association of short-term change in telomere length with cortical thickness changes and effects of mental training among healthy adults: a randomised clinical trial. *JAMA Network Open* 2019; 2 (9): e199687

McEwen, B.S. et al.: Stress effects on neuronal structure: hippocampus, amygdala, and prefrontal cortex. *Neuropsychopharmacology* 2016; 41 (1): 3–23

Michalsen, A. et al.: Iyengar yoga for distressed women: a 3-armed randomized controlled trial. *Evidence-based Complementary and Alternative Medicine* 2012; (467) 408727

Rapaport, M.H. et al.: A preliminary study of the effects of a single session of Swedish massage on hypothalamic-pituitary-adrenal and immune function in normal individuals. *Journal of Alternative and Complementary Medicine* 2010; 16 (10): 1079–1088

Reszka, E. et al.: Circadian genes in breast cancer. *Advances in Clinical Chemistry* 2016; 75: 53–70

Umfrage zum Weltglückstag 2019; Sinus Institut mit YouGov

Watson S.L. et al.: High-intensity resistance and impact training improves bone mineral density and physical function in postmenopausal women with osteopenia and osteoporosis: the LIFTMOR randomized controlled trial. *Journal of Bone and Mineral Research* 2018; 33 (2): 211–220

Wieland, L.S. et al.: Yoga treatment for chronic non-specific low back pain. *Cochrane Database Systematic Review* 2017, 1: CD010671

ONLINE RESOURCES

Deutsche Gesellschaft für Gynäkologie und Geburtshilfe e. V.
https://www.dggg.de
Deutsche Gesellschaft für Endokrinologie
https://www.endokrinologie.net
Deutsche Gesellschaft für Ernährung e. V.
https://www.dge.de
Bundesministerium für Umwelt, Naturschutz und nukleare Sicherheit
https://www.bmu.de
Robert Koch Institut
https://www.rki.de
World Health Organization (WHO)
https://www.who.int
Verbraucherzentrale
https://www.verbraucherzentrale.de
MBSR-MBCT-Verband
https://www.mbsr-verband.de
Australasian Menopause Society
https://www.menopause.org.au
British Menopause Society
https://thebms.org.uk
North American Menopause Society
https://www.menopause.org